Also by Ana Kolomeka

Wage Peace Between the Sexes (Spice Version): A Guide to Healthy and Wholesome Sensual Relationships for Youth

Escape the Apocalypse Through Future and Financial Planning (Hawaii Edition)

WAGE PEACE BETWEEN THE SEXES (SUGAR VERSION)

A GUIDE TO HEALTHY AND WHOLESOME SENSUAL RELATIONSHIPS FOR YOUTH

BY

ANA KOLOMEKA

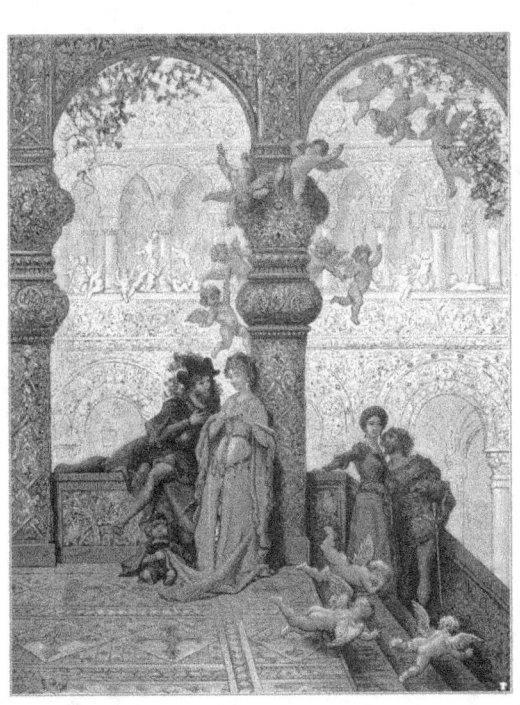

Publisher: Kahe Hohonu Na Wai Malie Press
Published in the United States of America

ISBN-13: 978-1506193434
ISBN-10: 1506193439

First Edition © 2015
Second Edition © 2015
Third Edition © 2016
Fourth Edition © 2017

Ana Kolomeka
P.O. Box 10192
Hilo, HI 96721
anakolomeka1@gmail.com

Comment as a guest on website:
http://hubpages.com/@anakolomeka

Like and comment on FaceBook:
https://www.facebook.com/pages/Truce-Between-the-Genders/1487075674912557?ref=hl

Dedicated with love to:

Mrs. Carol Diane Moses

Who taught me that Knowledge is Power

And led and inspired me by her excellent example.

THANK YOU!

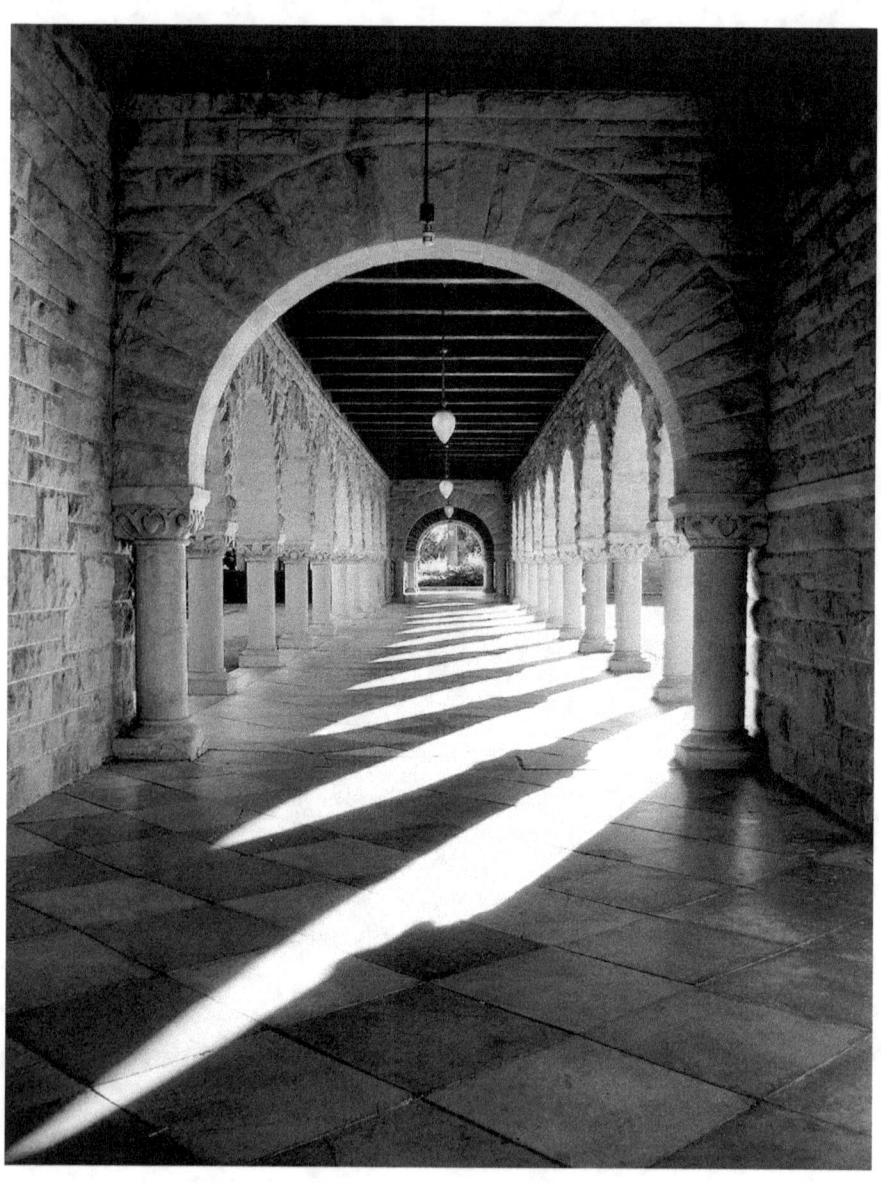

Table of Contents

INTRODUCTION

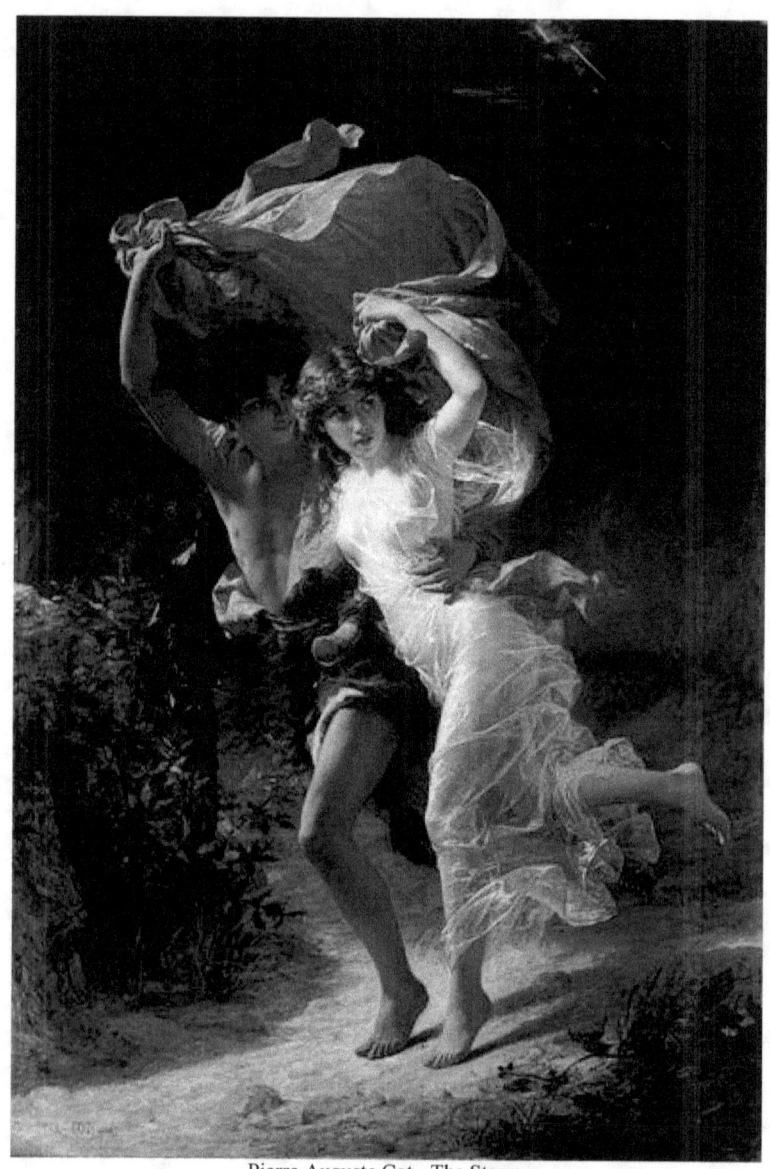

Pierre Auguste Cot - The Storm

My credentials (i.e., what WRITE do I have to RIGHT this book?)

Name: Ana Kolomeka

Age: Dark and evil times, which this book will dispel once enough people read it.

Sex: Sure, anytime! (Long as it's good)

Personal History: Rated NC17

Education: I have a BS, MS, and PhD. You know what BS stands for, right? Well, M.S. means More of the Same, and PhD is Piled Higher and Deeper.

Why I wrote this book: To wage peace between the sexes! What did you think?

Okay, let's get serious. My real inspiration comes from the fact that I grew up in the ghetto where the environment was basically ugly, ignorance was rampant, and men were something to be feared. Thanks to my favorite high school teacher, whom I've dedicated this book to, I was able to escape. I have since done considerable travelling, worked in a variety of fields, and had numerous experiences that have completely changed my view of the world. I have noticed that many people today have not been blessed with information I was lucky enough to obtain in high school. My purpose is to provide this education to those who lack caring teachers and the right surroundings, so they can take it upon themselves to become enlightened.

Some facts I point out in this book are:

Most men are not callous cheating criminals. They are perfectly capable of caring about women and children.

The divorce rate is a lot lower than the media portrays. It is calculated based on the number of marriages and divorces that occur in a given year; since there are typically half as many divorces, that's where you get the 50% statistic. A more accurate way of gauging is to count how many people have ever been divorced.

The biggest factor in divorce is *IGNORANCE*. Divorce rates vary according to how educated the partners are regarding relationships.

Physical beauty attracts, but quality of character is what holds a relationship together.

You attract what you are. Being the right person is every bit as important as finding the right person.

Sensual knowledge helps a relationships work; prudishness harms it.

About my credentials: this book is my thesis in an effort to obtain a PhD in the University of Hard Knocks. Yes I have a Bachelor's Degree, but the real learning comes outside of school. This is a collection of knowledge I've acquired from over a half century of observing and interacting with people, and studying a variety of cultures.

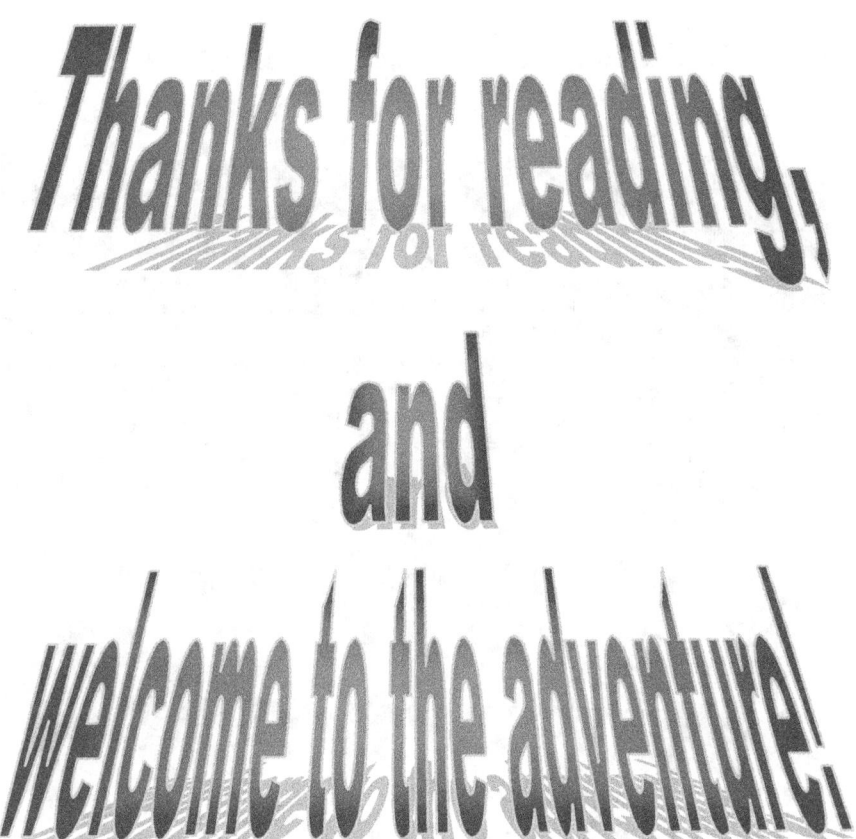

CHAPTER ONE

YES, YOU CAN BE AN ALPHA MALE / FEMALE!

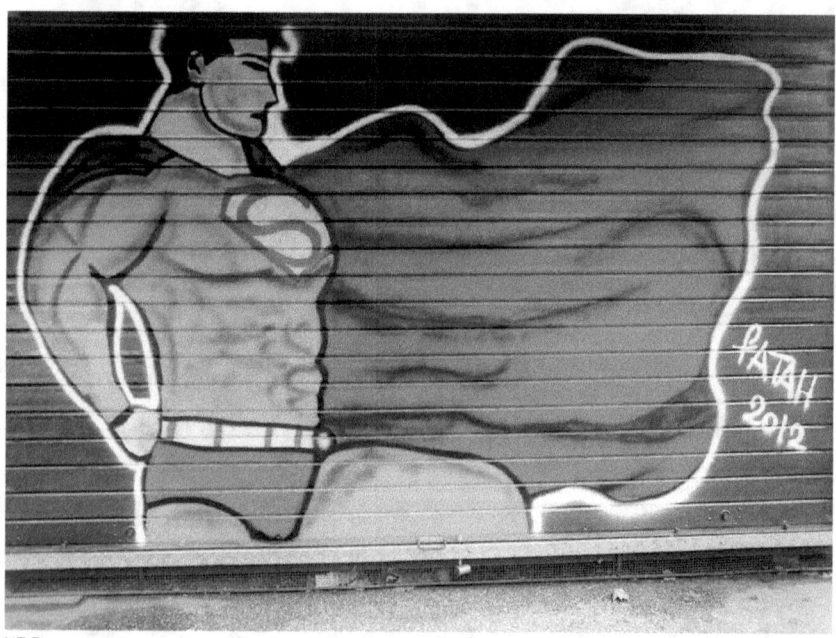

"No partner in a love relationship... should feel that he has to
give up an essential part of himself to make it viable."
~ May Sarton

Quiz:

Which of these statements are true, and which are false?

1) The title of this chapter refers to only a few select people

2) Alpha males and females are born, not made.

3) To be an alpha male / female, it is required to be tall and good looking, with athletic prowess.

4) Alpha males and females hog all the potential partners, leaving others bereft.

5) The best way to attract a boyfriend or girlfriend is to take an arrogant sour grapes attitude, acting like you don't need anybody.

6) Guys and girls basically don't like each other.

7) Most guys are criminals; some are just farther advanced than others.

8) Most girls are conniving gold diggers; some are just more successful than others.

9) Guys only care about getting into a girl's pants; girls only care about getting into a guy's wallet.

10) The surest way to be popular with the opposite sex is to be a master at psychological game playing.

Quiz Answers: All are false.

Why are you reading this book? Is it because you are truly curious about how the opposite gender thinks, and want to get to know them better? Girls; do guys scare you because you believe they are crude, unfeeling, violent? Guys; do you fear girls, thinking they're all greedy and manipulative?

We all know about alpha males and females. They attract like human magnets; often, their looks or wealth has little to do with their natural charisma. What is their secret to transcending the negative dating environment that is so pervasive throughout America?

The Day America Told the Truth, published in 1991, states that men and women basically don't like each other; men think of women as fussy cats, and women see men as boorish dogs. To verify this, a few years ago, I ran a poll on a social website; this is the result.

<u>Me:</u>	Men and boys - what do you like most about girls and women? What do you like the least? What I like best is that they're somehow easier to talk and relate to. What I like the least is when they're underhanded and backstabbing.
<u>Red:</u>	Well my type of girl is outgoing, understanding, sweet, cute, great sense of humor, not afraid to try, and loves to help. Girls I don't go for are the party girls that are kinda slutty, act bitchy, or are really plastic. Even if they're hot physically, actions and personality over weigh appearance.
<u>SettingSun:</u>	I like how friendly and understanding they are. How accepting and caring they are. Women seem to be more ready to stand up for what they believe in than guys some times. They are easier to talk to and relate to. They're not so quick to judge or laugh at you in a time of weakness, but they're a shoulder to cry on if needed (something most guys aren't good for

at all.) Those are just the good things, but that's all that matters. :-)

J. T: Smart women have qualities of modesty, honesty, tact, and obliging, polished manners. Stupid women are like stupid anything, but with the additional annoying air of expecting to get a free pass, just because they're women.

T. R.: The things that I like best about them is the fact that most of them are always willing to listen to whatever you have to say whether they can help or not. Another thing that I like is that they are usually easy to get along with and fun to be around. Some things that I don't like though is when they are very girly and just take forever to get ready to go out or just overdress for simple things to attract attention.

Alias: I think you fill find in this section most of the men don't like women at all lol.

Me: Girls and women – what do you like most about boys and men? What do you like the least? What I like the most is their sense of adventure; they're loads of fun. What I like the least is when they're criminals.

K. A.: I like it best when they are sensitive and can feel empathy for those less fortunate, and I absolutely despise it when they are easily upset and reveal a violent nature. =P Yes, I would not want to be with someone who is a criminal. =P.

Emma: What I like most is their sense of humor. I love laughing and making other laugh, and if a guy has that in common then we'll always have fun.   I like the adventurous and competitive side, too. :) Least is temper or aggression. Sometimes the temper is sparked

15

from jealousy but I like when a guy is just chill.

Ann: Most – They're funny and playful. Least – If they're violent.

E. L.: I like that they have d**ks. I dislike that they are d**ks.

2B or not 2B   I like when they're funny.

Based on this survey, I think it's safe to say men and women do like each other as a rule; they just have difficulty relating to the opposite gender, because of lack of knowledge or belief in circulating myths. Some may harbor resentment because of bad experiences, in which case they need counseling to overcome this.

The bottom line is this: If you're going to be an alpha male or female, you have to *genuinely like the opposite sex*. If you do, the rest will come naturally. If you don't, nothing else will matter – because they will sense that, and you will either repel them, or attract negative types. The way to learn to like them is to focus on their positive traits. Make a list of what you like best about the opposite sex, and read it every day. As for their negative attributes, learn what situations promote those, and avoid them. Contrary to what the media may have you believe, most people are inherently good; they are far more interested in living positive lives than destroying those of others. The world is also improving; every day, we come up with cures for diseases and better ways of doing basic tasks through technology. That's why you're able to read this in various formats, including ebook; centuries ago, you would have been lucky to even get an education, and then you would have needed your wealthy parents to provide you with this in hardcover. Even then, most of the information in here would not have been available!

So let's say you truly like the opposite gender. Now what?

Here are some traits for guys to develop:

Though most animals gain status by brawling over females, that is not necessary among humans; being a troublemaking bully actually hurts one's chances. Alpha Males do not start fights; they end them. They have good battle skills, but they use them for

16

defense, not to start trouble. Listed below are three main ways to become an Alpha Male.

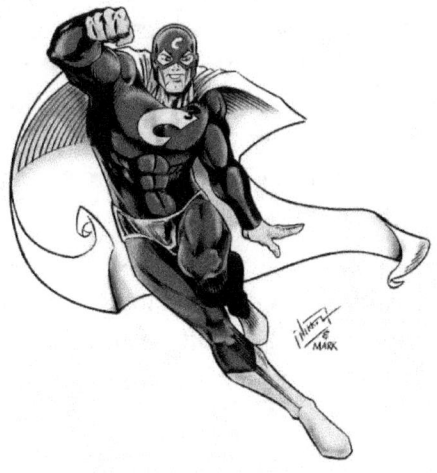

Alpha Male

1) <u>Look the part</u>. You don't have to be built like Mr. Universe, but you should look as if you care about your health. Exercise on a regular basis. The best way to stay on track with a program is to engage in your favorite sport, and cross train for it. Include a healthy diet with your regime. Good grooming is also necessary; be neat and clean in your appearance, and wear clothing that fits the occasion, rather than being too formal or casual. Also, watch your body language. Look people in the eye when you talk with them, sit and stand straight, and speak in a normal tone of voice, neither too dominant nor passive.

2) <u>Be a leader</u>. Becoming an Alpha Male isn't about dominating, rather, it's being confident enough to naturally lead others. The best way to achieve this is to educate yourself; the broader your knowledge base, the greater your leadership chances. Realize that education doesn't end when you graduate from school, it continues throughout life. Also, it is very important to listen to your followers, so you know how best to meet their needs. True leaders are chosen, so your chances depend

17

on your ability to be of service to others. Girls are naturally drawn to leaders, but being an emotionally abusive womanizer is a surefire way to run them off; the only ones who will stay are the neurotics. To attract and keep emotionally healthy girls, treat them well; be chivalrous, and be honest regarding your intentions, rather than falsely stringing them along. When you choose a girlfriend, remain faithful to her, and consider her needs first.

3) <u>Be confident enough to take chances</u>. The Alpha Male isn't afraid to make mistakes. He knows that's how people learn. If he makes a mistake in public, he has the confidence and sense of humor to laugh and try again. There is something highly attractive about a guy who is willing to take risks. Such a guy also tends to have the most successes.

Here are qualities for girls to develop:

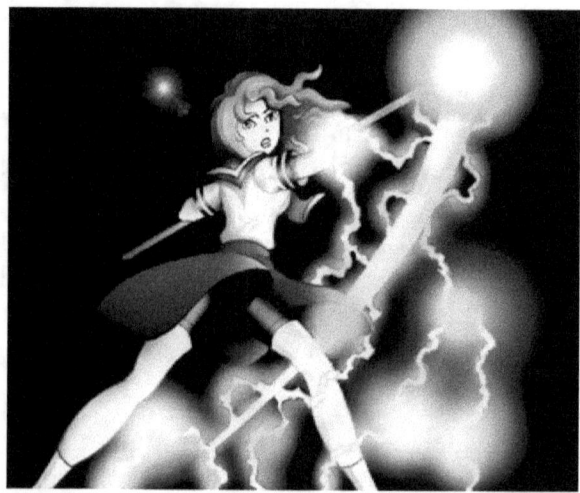

Alpha Female

1) <u>Watch your appearance</u>. Like guys, it is best to be physically fit and as healthy as possible; it shows you care about yourself, leading others to care about you. Fashion wise, people tend to judge girls more harshly than guys, so how you dress is important too – however, it is best to go for a style that is unique and comfortable,

rather than stressing to wear the latest, most expensive fashions. Wear only minimal makeup, and comfortable shoes (your feet will thank you later, when you avoid permanently curled-up toes!). Carrying yourself with a certain brash attitude will lead others to regard you as an Alpha Female.

2) <u>Develop a confident, sure personality</u>. Many girls nitpick at themselves, complaining about their weight or looks; they may constantly change their opinions based on what they believe to be popular; or they lack independence and cling too tightly to guys. Some will clutch any guy who gives them the time of day! Being comfortable in your own skin not only helps you be better company, it makes you downright sexy, too. Also, rather than use manipulation to win a guy, seek to understand a wide array of them, making friends with them and truly caring. Another important factor is to fully enjoy the life you lead. Laugh out loud, enjoy your favorite activities whenever you can, eat all you want and exercise the calories off. This will add more to an Alpha aura than virtually anything else.

3) <u>Have a generous spirit</u>. Avoid being suspicious, especially viewing other girls as competition. Realize that there is enough of everything for everyone, and love freely. The idea that Alpha Females are bitchy is a myth; the true ones attract others and achieve leadership through love, not jealousy and control. When guys gather around you, invite other girls along to share the joy. Encourage girls to develop themselves and meet great guys. The likelihood of another girl stealing your boyfriend from you is not that great, and even if it happened, that says unsavory things about him; do you really want a guy so easily taken?

As you see, the requirements for being an Alpha Male and Alpha Female are very similar. Guys and girls are actually more alike than different; we have pretty much the same desires, and love and hurt the same.

19

So what is the real difference between guys and girls? Here is a list:

Women live longer than men, but the quality of those extra years is more likely to be poor.

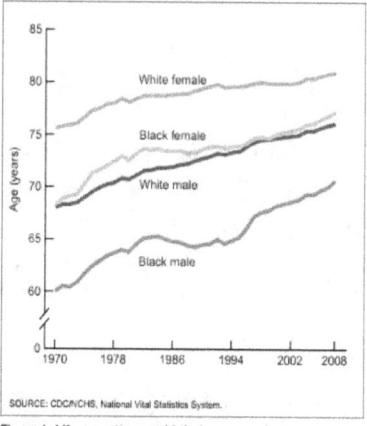

Figure 1. Life expectancy at birth, by race and sex: United States, 1970–2008

(Actually, Asian women have the longest life expectancy, and Native American men from South Dakota the lowest.)

That's why the nursing home population is overwhelmingly female. As a general rule, men burn out; women fade away.

Physically, men are stronger and faster, while women are more flexible and better at endurance.

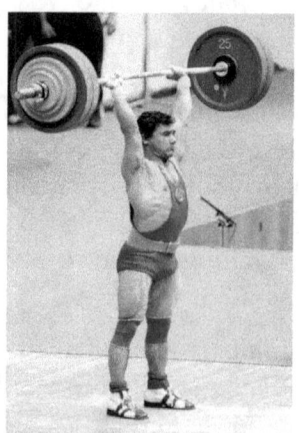
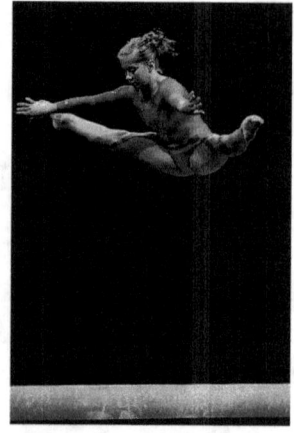

Once, a boyfriend took me to Yosemite. Even though he's a couch potato, he raced up the trail, leaving me in the dust. Yet that night, he was worn out, while I felt fine, even though I'd hiked the same distance.

Women gain weight more easily than men, because their bodies have more fat composition, whereas men have more muscle. However health wise, women can get away with more extra poundage than men. That is because women put weight on their hips, whereas men wear it above their waists, closer to the heart. Ever heard the saying, "Men are apples; women are pears"? That's what that means.

Regarding physical changes growing old, men are more likely to turn gray or lose their hair altogether; women are more likely to wrinkle.

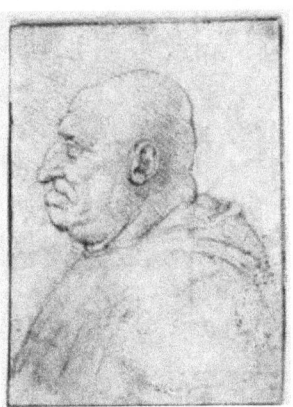 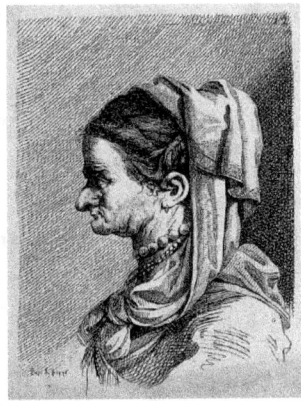

Women age suddenly, especially after menopause; men age more gradually, and are more likely to take on female characteristics. This is all due to hormones.

Women's ability to conceive reduces after 35, resulting in complete infertility after menopause. A man can always father a baby, but if he is past 50, the child is more likely to become schizophrenic.

Men are more slated to be criminals, but they're also more inclined to be heroes.

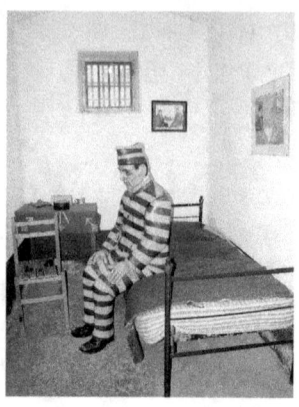 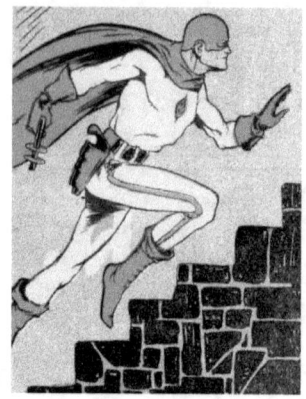

Check out the annals of history; most famous people, good and evil, are men. However, the majority of men are good, and even scuzzy-looking ones can surprise you with positive traits. Most women are good too, but if she is evil, she hides it better; as a result, she is more likely to get away with it, while men are more prone to serving sentences for crimes they didn't commit. For girls who are attracted to villains, or want to perpetuate that lifestyle themselves, bear in mind the criminal world is extremely sexist. Most females there either are exploited, working in dangerous low-level occupations such as streetwalking, or they merely aid and abet, depending on their boyfriends for their needs. Few achieve leadership status of any kind.

NOW FOR THE BIG QUESTION. WHAT DO GIRLS WANT???

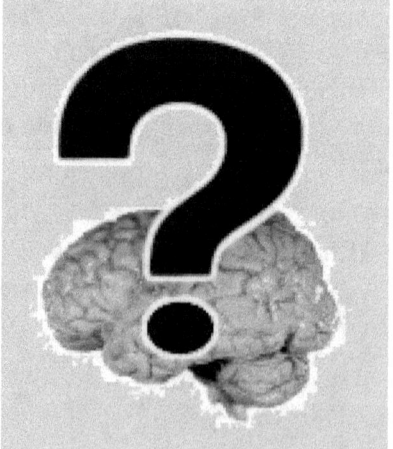

Believe it or not, girls aren't that complex (well some are, but you can find one who isn't). Most want a guy who respects girls in general and her in particular. Being chivalrous is still appreciated by most; anyone who rudely rejects such gestures should be avoided, anyway. Girls want someone who is mature, responsible, and stable. Being clean and neat in appearance is also necessary, because that displays how a guy feels about himself. Good courtship involves being attentive, emotionally involved, and creative; continually, think of new ways to express how you feel, and come up with novel ideas for dates. Girls generally prefer guys to take the lead in a relationship, and be financially secure.

WE HAVE TO BE FAIR, HERE. WHAT DO GUYS LOOK FOR IN A GIRL?

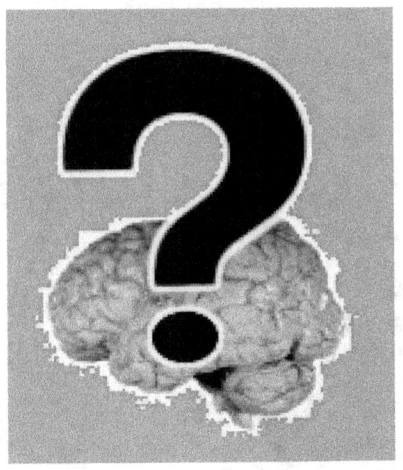

Confidence is a *HUGE* factor. Few things turn guys off more than constant apprehension and jealousy. Definitely, never inflict on him the dreaded question, "Honey, do I look fat?" (Guys; if a girl says that to you, respond with, "Honey, do I look stupid?") Other qualities guys appreciate in a girl are honesty, a sense of humor, intelligence, playfulness, spontaneity, and the ability to relax in the relationship. Though guys often like to treat their girlfriends like princesses, they prefer someone who is undemanding and non-materialistic. They find it highly commendable if she is independent enough to allow him time with his buddies, pursuing their favorite sports and hobbies. They like girls who are sensual, and emotionally supportive without being suffocating.

Contrary to popular belief, most guys are not sluts; they are perfectly capable of caring about their girlfriends and remaining faithful to them. Players usually are easy to spot; in fact, many will come right out and tell you. What gets a girl into trouble is when she tries to change him, or convinces herself that he will make an exception for her if he loves her enough. In reality, being in love does not alter one's basic character; poor self-esteem and lack of respect for the opposite sex remain factors in how he treats others. (A prime example is Whitney Houston and Bobby Brown's marriage. She was the love of his life, but that didn't keep him from abusing her.) When you spot a player, it is best to accept him for what he is, and let him associate with other swingers while you find someone who will be true to you (unless you're a swinger yourself, of course – but that's a topic for another book).

As a general rule, girls go for professions while guys are attracted by looks.

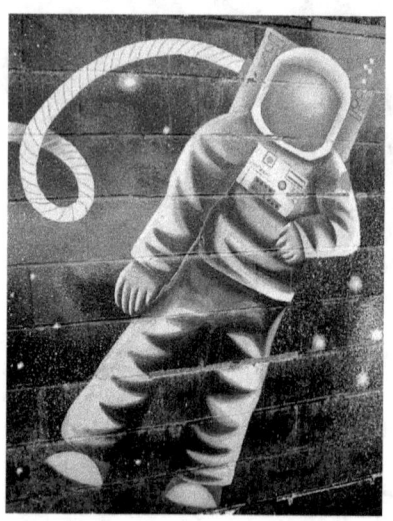
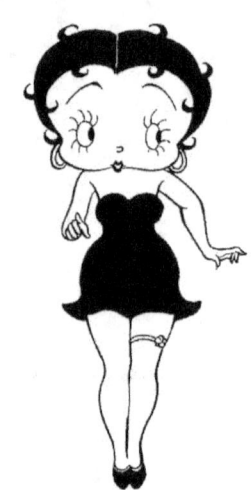

Guys are turned on by sight; girls by situations. It is common for them to be drawn to those who closely resemble the opposite gender parent, which presents a problem for those who come from a dysfunctional home. Self-knowledge and counseling can go a long way for resolving such matters.

Now that we've set these issues straight, let's develop a healthy, positive attitude towards the opposite gender, appreciate each other, and celebrate our differences! These are the best strategies for attracting an ideal mate, and waging peace between the sexes.

One final note: though this book is primarily aimed at heterosexuals, homosexuals of either gender can benefit from it as well.

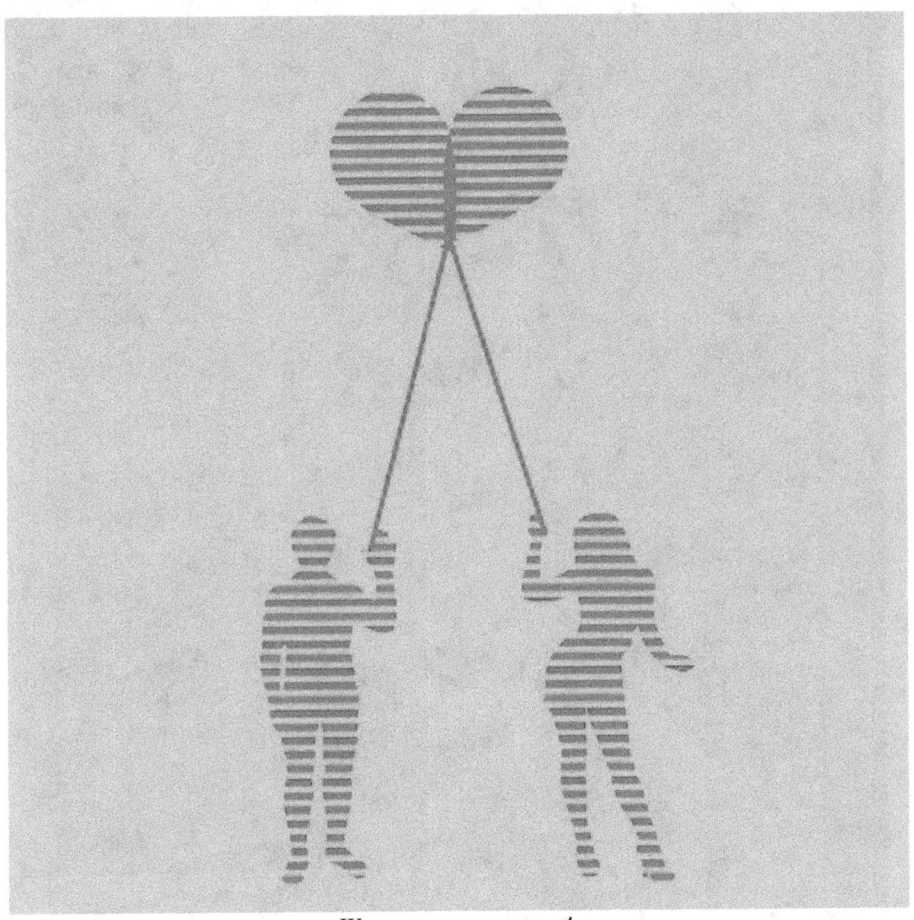

Wage peace, not war!

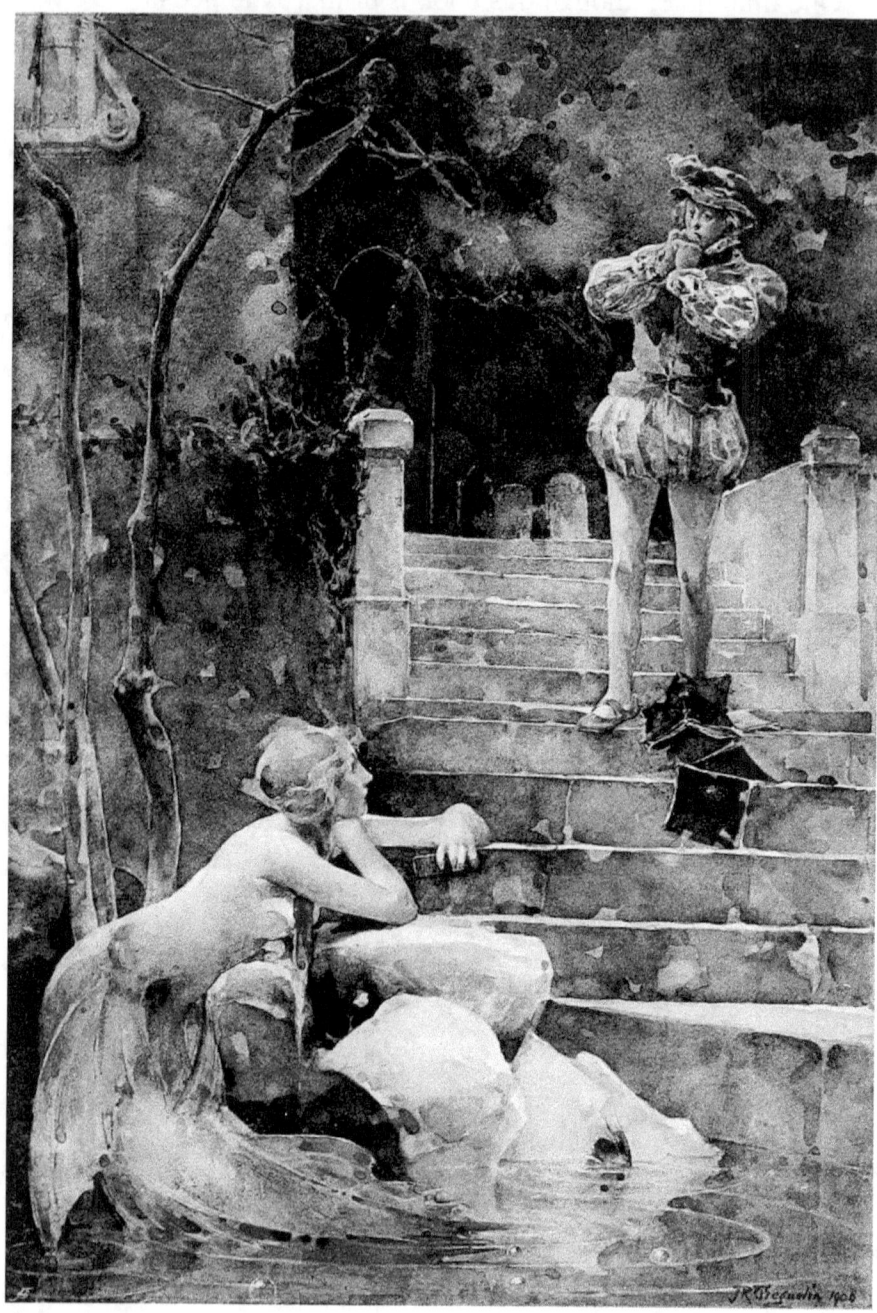

Activity:

1) What do you like about people of your gender? What do you dislike?

2) What do you like about members of the opposite gender? What do you dislike?

3) Describe the ideal person of your gender, using the character template from this website:

   http://imaginingsofacreativewriter.blogspot.com/2012/05/character-profile-sheet.html

   How well do you fit this description?

4) Now, describe the ideal person of the opposite gender using the same template.

   Do you know anyone who fits this description?

CHAPTER TWO

ALL THE GOOD ONES ARE TAKEN – *REALLY?*

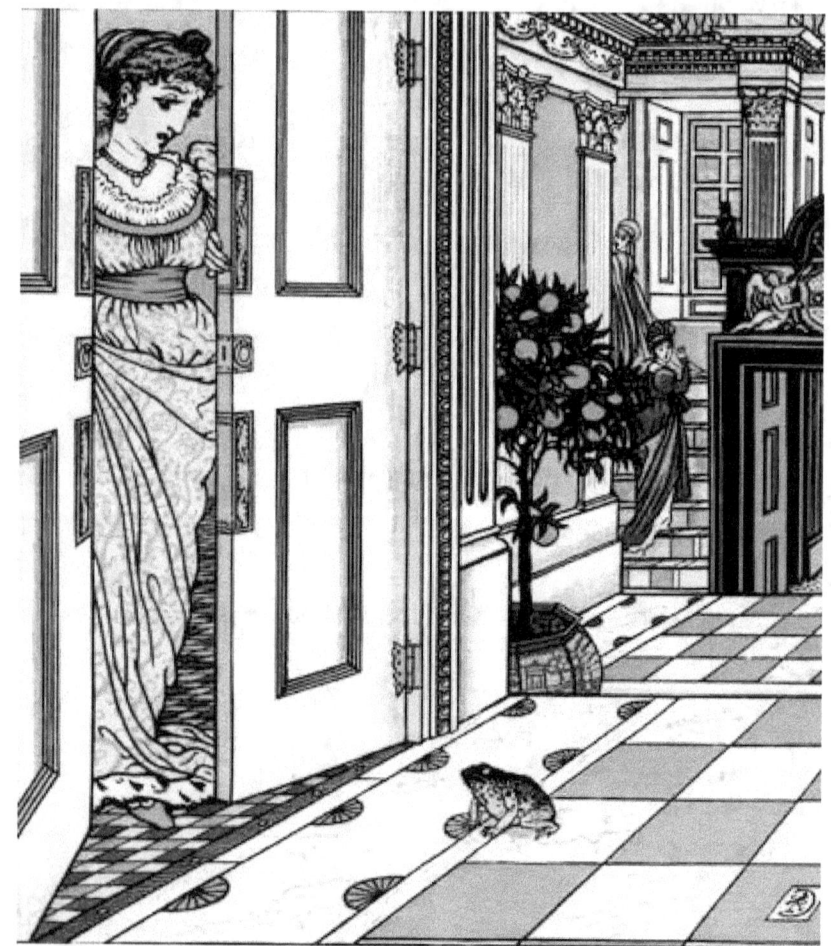

"In order to meet a handsome prince, you have to kiss a lot of frogs!"
~ from *The Frog Prince*

Put on the Hot Seat:

Which of these statements are true, and which are false?

1) When looking for a relationship, rather than zeroing in on just one person, it is best to reach out to several people, even if they're not a potential partner.

2) There is a lot you can do to liven your school's social scene, if it's dead.

3) It is possible to have a great time on a date without involving sex, alcohol, or drugs.

4) It is best to wait until a relationship has existed several months, or even a year, before having sex.

5) Sex, alcohol, and drugs, rather than enhance a date or relationship, can actually ruin both.

6) Meeting great guys and girls is actually not as hard as the media would have you believe. Multiple venues exist.

7) You cannot truly fall in love at first sight; you must know the other person in order to truly love him or her.

8) Dating services are unnecessary if you make enough of an effort to join societies and clubs and remain active in them.

9) Dates don't have to be expensive to be fun.

10) The purpose of dating is to get to know one another, rather than impress each other.

Answers: All are true.

Since you're still in school, you have an advantage for potential good relationships; simply take part in as many social activities as possible, making a point of reaching out to others in the process. Even then though, much prevents an educational institution from being an ideal place; high school students are often too immature to handle even themselves, let alone a partner, and those in college are busy training for a career.

For adults no longer in academia, meeting someone for a relationship can be a real problem. They have more freedom to seek a mate; however, optimal meeting places are difficult to find. Bars and nightclubs often lead to shallow relationships at best, and alcoholics, even axe murderers, at worst. Hence the age-old question: where do you meet great guys / girls? Listed below are some ideas. You can use these venues even while you're in school; this is a good idea if your campus has few social activities, or a small student body.

WHERE TO MEET GREAT GIRLS

Yoga / Ballet / Zumba exercise

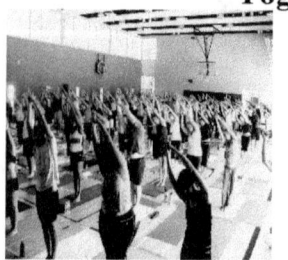 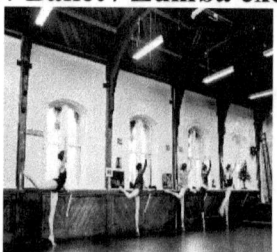 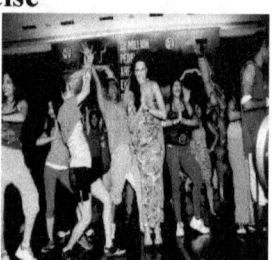

These tend to be overwhelmingly female; however, there's no need for a guy to feel out of place here, since showing his sensitive side will attract girls big time. It is best to socialize after class. You can strike up a casual conversation, and ask her – or several others – out for sodas and shakes.

Cooking courses

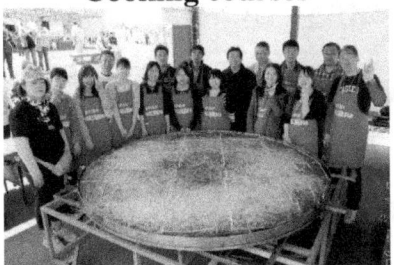

Though this has traditionally been a woman's role, many of the world's best chefs are male, so you'll fit in here.

Acting

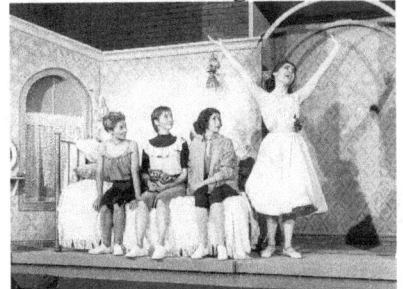

Though 75% of Hollywood roles go to men, most aspiring actors are female. You will have no shortage here!

Foreign language studies

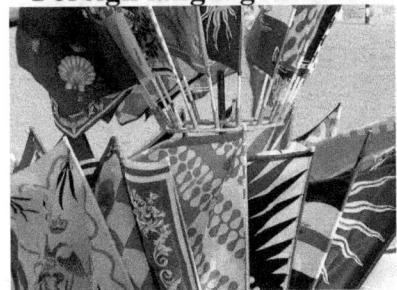

These attract girls who enjoy travelling. Perhaps this could lead to shared adventures.

Dance classes

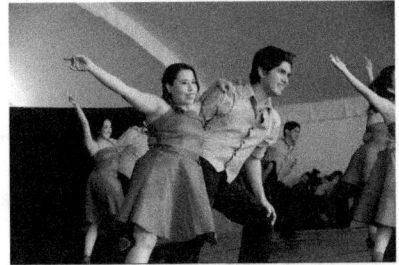

Girls love to dance, and often there's a gender imbalance, making it a great place for guys to meet them. Square, ballroom and swing are a sure bet. If you're a great dancer, you'll have girls fighting over you.

Art gallery exhibits

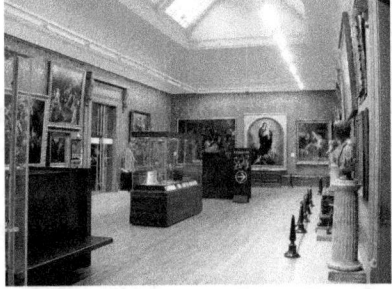

Girls also tend to love fine art.

Tennis Courts

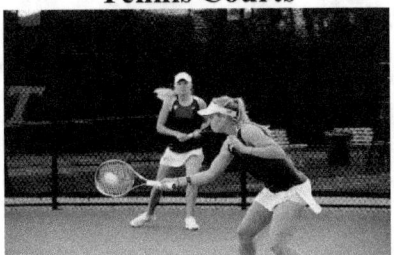

In recent decades, women have dominated the tennis world.

WHERE TO MEET GREAT GUYS

Sports clubs

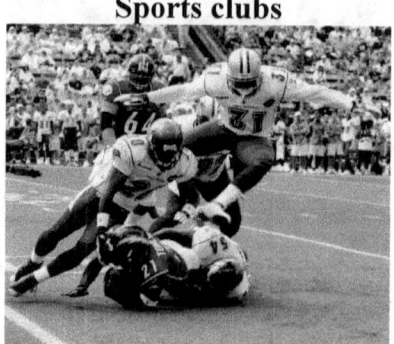

Check out groups and teams in your area. Ski and snowboard clubs tend to be mostly male; so do surfing groups. Also, some cities have teams that play basketball, football, and baseball. If you don't want to actually participate in the sport, offer to work at organizing events, and cook for them.

Advance math class, or a computer programming course

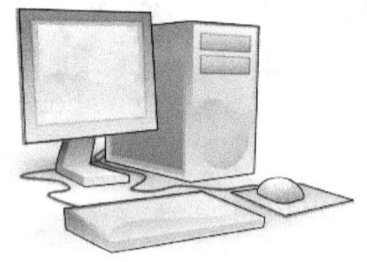

These can be found at reasonable prices at a local community college. If you personally use spreadsheets, learning macros can increase your skills.

Auto shop schools

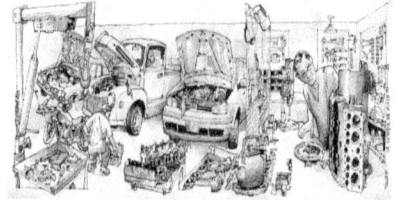

You can take a course yourself, get a clerical job there, or simply hang out and provide great food for the students.

Skate parks

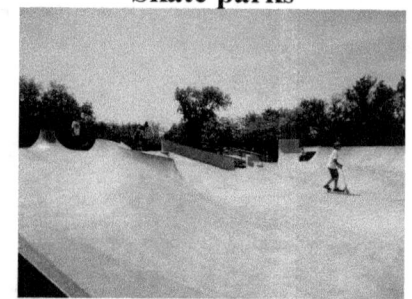

The skateboarding world is dominated by guys.

Music stores

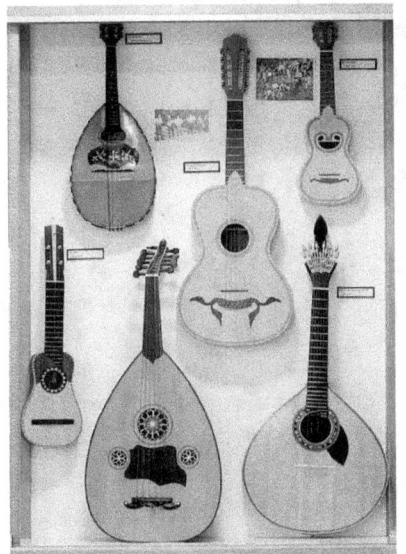

Guys enjoy shopping for audio equipment and instruments. The best stores are those that advertise for band members. You can join a band yourself, or make a habit of buying guitar strings, recorded music, and other things there.

Sailing clubs, and maritime navigating courses

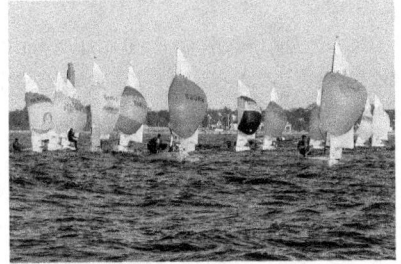

Guys enjoy sailing and motor boating as well.

Astronomy

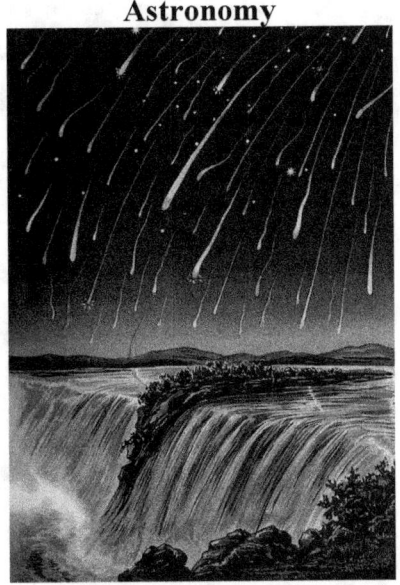

This science field also has a high ratio of guys, and it is fascinating besides. You can both enjoy a date studying the night sky sometime.

Golf courses

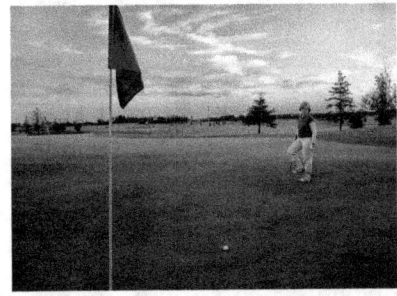

Generally, the men you meet here will be older with some wealth (so take this route if you're over 18, and go for guys who are not too much older than you). If you have considerable means yourself, you could join a golf or country club.

Rock climbing / batting cage / indoor skiing-snowboarding center.

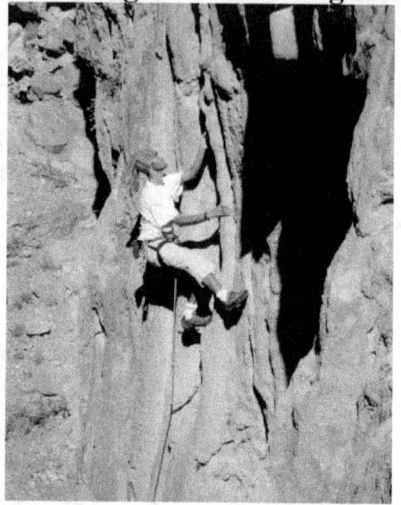

Since guys are very much into these sports, you'll meet plenty of them here.

WHERE TO MEET BOTH

Coffee shops / bookstores

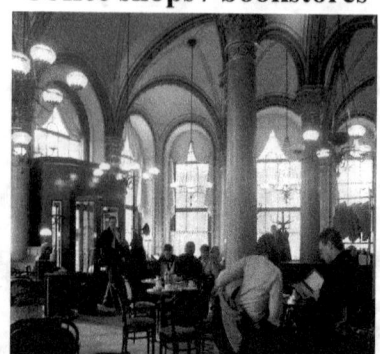

Church

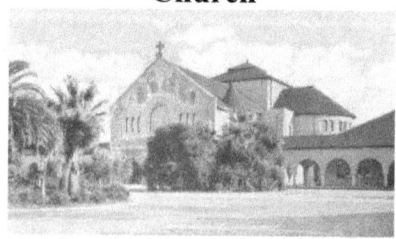

Stanford Memorial Church

Educated people are drawn to such places. You can enjoy a chai latte while discussing what the other is reading, the latest news and trends, etc.

A large active membership comprising people of all ages is a good bet. Obviously, avoid the ones consisting almost exclusively of little children and the elderly.

Skating rinks

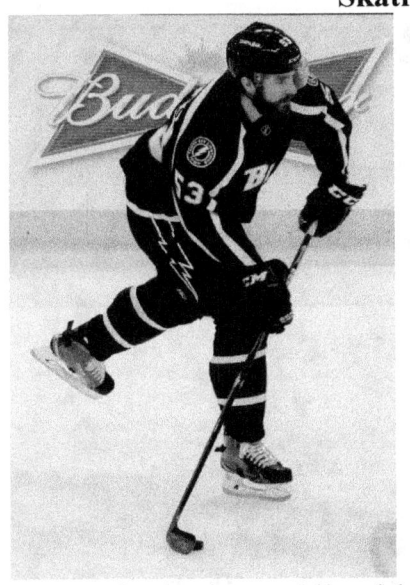
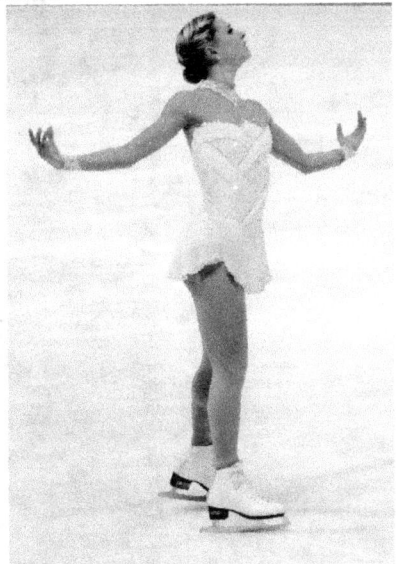

Guys go for hockey, while girls prefer figure skating. It's a great opportunity for them to get together after class.

Ecology clubs

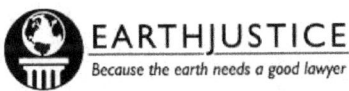

Groups like the Sierra Club, where they're working to save the environment, draws caring people. Working towards a shared cause is a great way to have something in common.

Community service

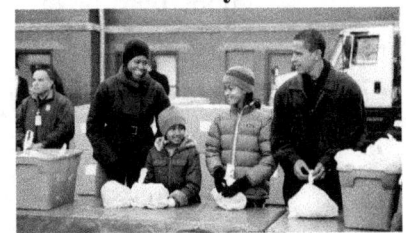

These, like ecology clubs, also attract caring individuals. You can get to know each other while working on a worthy project you both believe in. **Meetup.com** lists a variety of interest-based associations in your local area.

College cafeterias

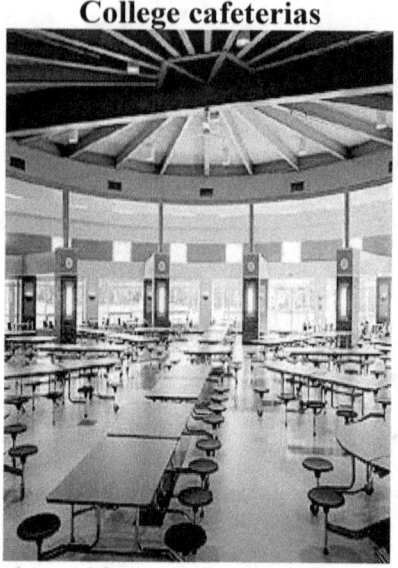

This is best if you're already a college student. It can be tricky striking up a conversation, since you're with a stranger knowing nothing about him or her; joining a campus club or taking a class can make the process easier.

PARTIES GIVEN BY FRIENDS

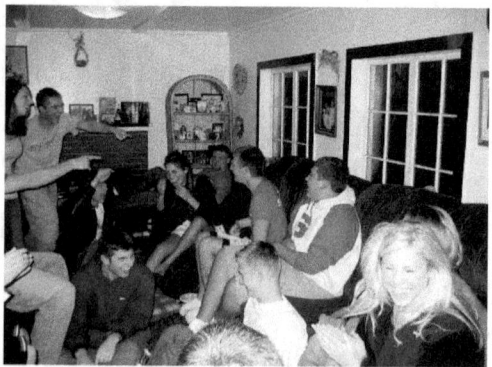

This can be the best way to meet someone - and also the worst. The more popular you are, the more likely you will meet a partner through friends; but the quality of such a person depends on the type of company you surround yourself with.

Perhaps you're the friend hosting the party. How do you prevent it from being a flop? Here are some games that have proven to be excellent mixers.

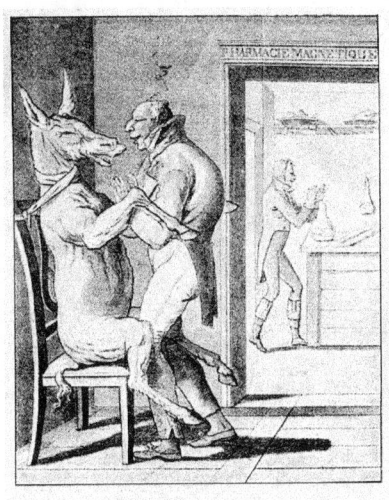

NOS FACULTÉS SONT EN RAPPORT. AQUATINT

Smart Ass: This game calls for 2 to 8 players. First, sort the cards according to the four categories. The yellow side of the card should be played first. The starting player rolls the die, chooses a card according to its category, and reads the 10 clues on there while the others try to guess the correct answer. The one who calls it out first moves his or her token along the board, and gets to be "it" next. The first player to reach the end of the board wins.

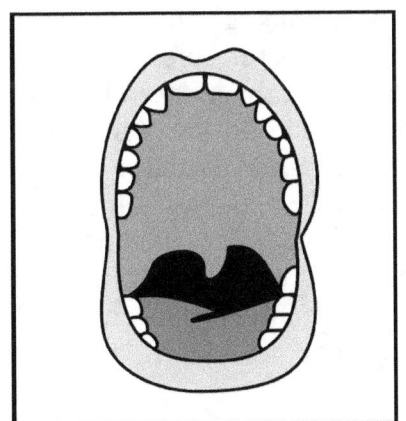

Say Anything. You will need 3 to 8 players; ideally, people you know well. One person draws a card, and reads the question on it. A typical question is one like, "In your opinion, what is the greatest movie ever made?" The others write their responses on white boards, and the player secretly chooses the answer he or she likes best. Everyone who correctly guessed the answer that was chosen gets a point. The one with the most points at the end of the game wins.

<u>Loaded Questions</u>. The ideal number of players is 3 to 6. The 1st player rolls the die, moves the token to that place on the board, and reads the corresponding card question. The others write the answer and pass it to the player, who guesses who wrote what answer.

These games can all be found on Amazon.com. <u>Smart Ass:</u> http://www.   amazon.com/University-Games-1360-Smart-Ass/dp/ B000NP4832 . <u>Say Anything:</u> http://www.amazon.com/s/ref=nb _sb_noss_2?url=search-alias%3   Dtoys-and-games&   field-keywords=Say+Anything . <u>Loaded Questions:</u> http:// www amazon.com   /s/ref=nb_sb_noss_2?url=search-alias%3Dtoys-and-games& field-keywords=Loaded+ Questions&rh=n%3A165793011 %2Ck%3ALoaded+ Questions .

Another idea besides games is holding a dance. Ballroom and swing dance lessons will be a real asset here; though guys have traditionally led in dancing, those who have taken lessons can lead for those who haven't. Also, you can do line dancing or Zumba, using videos as a guide. You can also find someone who knows how to teach circle mixers; in this case, couples dance in a circle, changing partners throughout. Though it is traditionally done to Irish jigs and reels, any type of music in 6/8 or 4/4 time will do; just set up the player to make it last 15 minutes or longer. Or hire a band from your school to play at your party!

INTERNET DATING

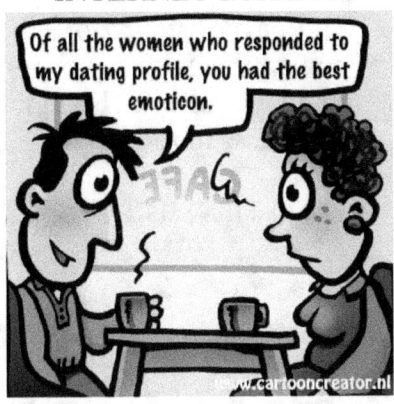

I will be blunt here; internet dating is not for high school students. It's tough enough for experienced adults to navigate; kids new to the dating scene and relationships have enough to deal with without the added burdens of the internet. There are nearly a thousand sites dedicated exclusively to matching couples; they cater to every imaginable basis such as age, race, economic status, sexual orientation, career, and hobby interests. It is even possible to "date" people who live in other countries, using Skype to communicate face to face. In addition most social media sites such as FaceBook, Twitter, or Yelp, offer services. However, scams abound; many dating sites will gladly take your money, then not offer what they promised. Some are phishing venues, designed to use your personal information to steal your identity; others are a front for prostitution. Dating sites can also be an ideal way for criminals to find unwary victims. Since navigating such a huge array of choices can be daunting, it is best to date people you actually know, and who can be screened by your parents. Most reputable sites require participants to be at least 18 years of age, so membership wouldn't be available to the majority of high school students, anyway. If your home town doesn't have enough social activities or accessible potential mates, make a point of taking vacations to more suitable places and keep in touch with whoever you meet there.

Ultimately the most successful people in the dating game are those with good social skills. Just as important as making connections – if not more so – is maintaining them. Be friendly with everyone; rather than focusing on one person, talk with lots of

39

people, regardless of whether or not they're dating material. Someone unsuitable could have a sibling or other relative, or know someone you could be compatible with.

Remember, it's a numbers game. The more sheer volume you get, the more likely your success in finding the Right One.

DATING IDEAS

Rapunzel enjoys a secret rendezvous with the prince

Nowadays, a lot of people make the mistake of having sex too soon in the relationship. Some even do it on the first date! The pitfalls to this are many; since you don't know the person very well, you have no idea if they will abuse your vulnerabilities, have sexually transmitted diseases, or particularly nasty faults like violence. A girl could deceive a guy about being on birth control and get pregnant in an effort to trap him. These are only a few examples of what could go wrong, but the bottom line is, after having sex, you may discover certain things about that person which, if you'd known earlier, you wouldn't have given him or her the time of day!

Sex is best enjoyed with someone you know and can fully trust. Here are ten ideas for dates that don't involve sex. This list is by no means exhaustive.

Go out for sodas, or shakes.

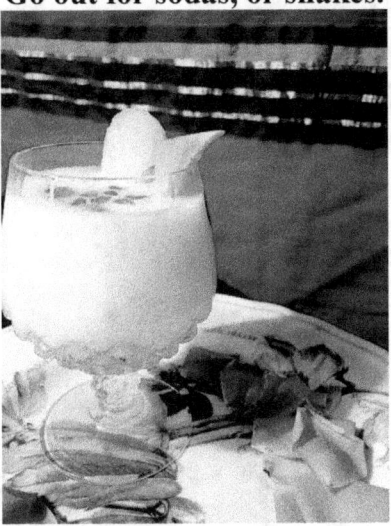

This is ideal for people who are getting together for the first time. Be sure to bring a mental list of topics to discuss. If you run short on ideas, coffee shops usually have books and newspapers the two of you can browse.

Go to a movie

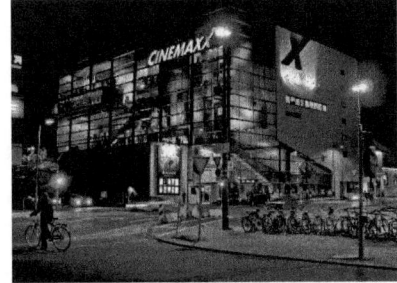

The two of you can discuss it afterwards

Go to a school dance

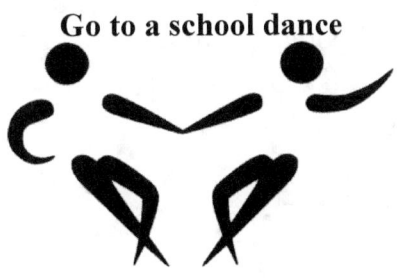

If you took lessons, you can use the moves you learned there to wow the kids.

41

Go bowling / play golf

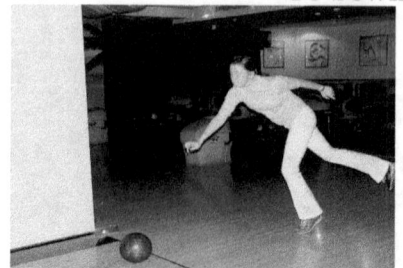 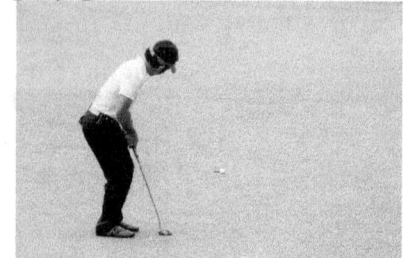

You can compete and still be comrades.

Go ice skating / roller-blading

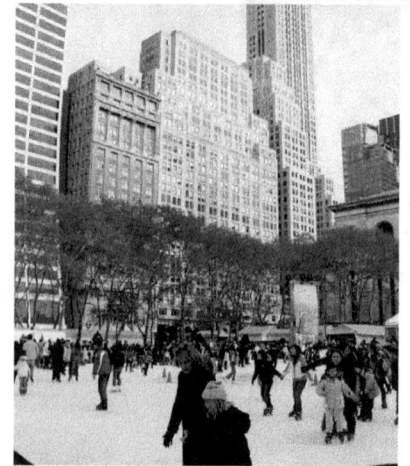 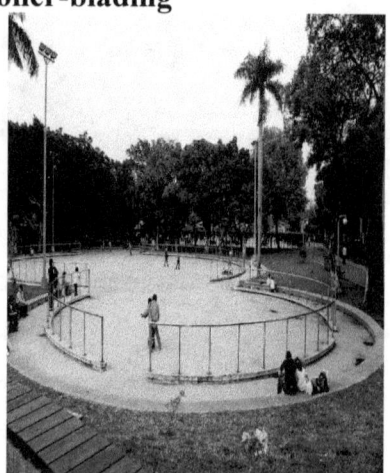

In some places, people still meet at skating rinks. Also, you can incorporate ballroom / swing dance moves into this medium.

Go on group hikes / attend a beach party with friends

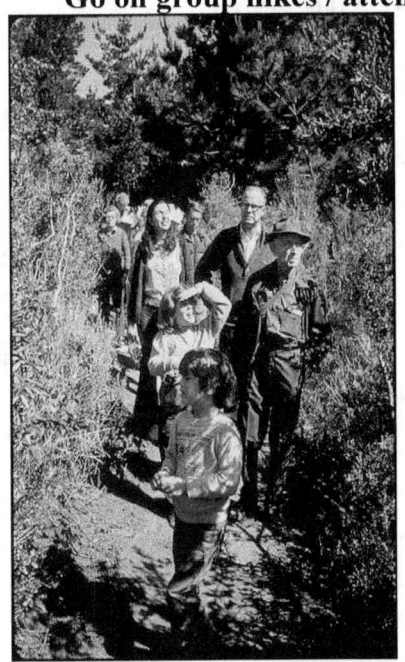
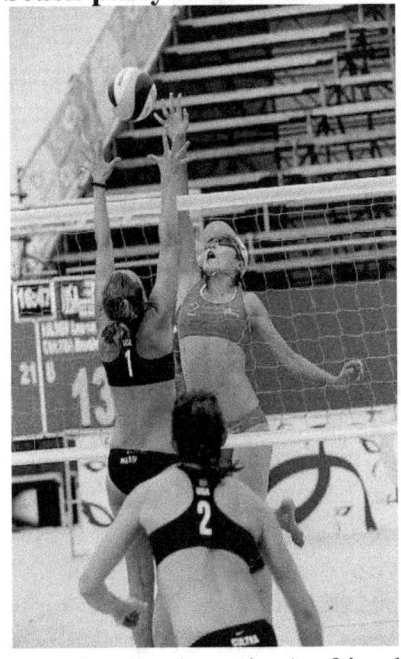

Group activities are ideal for getting to know the other's friends. You can see how well you fit into each other's communities; important if you're to share lives.

Go skiing / snowboarding

Take a simple walk in the park

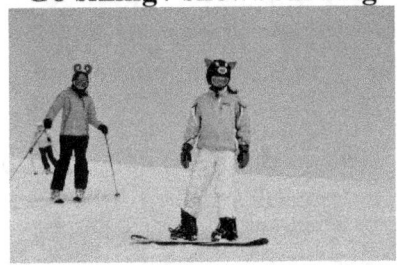
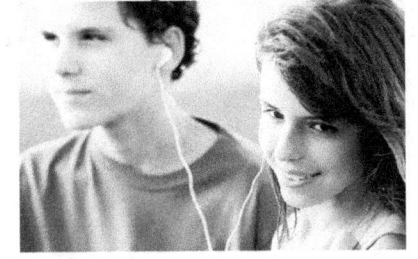

Sharing a sport is a great way to get to know one another, and keep in good physical shape at the same time (in Hawaii, you can do this on Mauna Kea).

In some ways, this could be the best date of all. With nothing distracting you, you can truly get to know one another.

Note I didn't include alcohol and drugs in any of these ideas. The drinking age nationwide is 21, and drugs are illegal, for good reason; using them can lead to poor judgment, bringing about negative situations such as date rape, DUI convictions, and health problems that can impact one for life. Though jokes about drunkenness and debauchery abound, nothing ruins the potential of a good relationship like behaving that way on a date.

Who should pay on dates? In the past, it was the guy, since as adults the man's role was to be the breadwinner, while women rarely worked outside the house. Now this issue is newly complex, with the advent of women having careers, people delaying marriage long after they graduate from school, and both husband and wife working to afford the outrageously expensive rents for apartments in prosperous locations. However, since men on average earn 25% more than women, and women are more likely to take time off work to care for children and aging relatives, it is still preferred that the man bear most of the costs of dating. The current custom is that the guy usually covers all the outlay for the first date; afterwards, the girl should offer to help out. For example, if they see a movie, he buys the tickets while she pays for the popcorn. Some guys like to always treat their girls; that should be respected. Going Dutch, where each person pays his or her own tab, is not a good idea, since it kills the spirit; it is better to share. Of course make sure you only go on dates you can afford; the girl should not gouge the guy, and neither should the guy overextend himself. If he does so as an attempt to impress her, it won't work; it will only make him look irresponsible. If he's trying to give her a guilt trip so she will have sex with him, he risks committing date rape (more about that in the next chapter).

It is also fine for a girl to ask a guy for a date; she can do so by casually stating she has two passes to a cool event in town, and would he be interested in joining her? As a rule, whoever asks for the date pays for it.

Enjoying an active, vibrant social life which eventually leads to meeting the Right One is not terribly difficult. All it takes is knowledge, and the wisdom to apply it.

Cause a Commotion:

1. Is the social scene dead at your school? If so, what can *YOU* do to turn things around? Get together with some teachers and fellow students, to brain storm ideas. A few tips; if your school is small, you can join up with other schools to enlarge your social pool. You can poll other students, and start interest clubs that way. Also, search the web for simple line dances, done both as singles and as couples; next time the school hosts a dance, have someone teach them to everyone there.

2. If the social scene is good at your school, join 3 clubs and remain active in them.

3. Make a long list of members of the opposite sex that go to your school. Make a point of talking to each one, and find out 3 facts about each of them. Continually reach out to others, whether or not they make potential dates. This may be painful to some, but good social skills are *VITAL* in being successful in life. Keep practicing; in time, it gets easier.

4. Describe, in detail, your version of the ideal date that doesn't involve sex, drugs or alcohol. Compare your response with others.

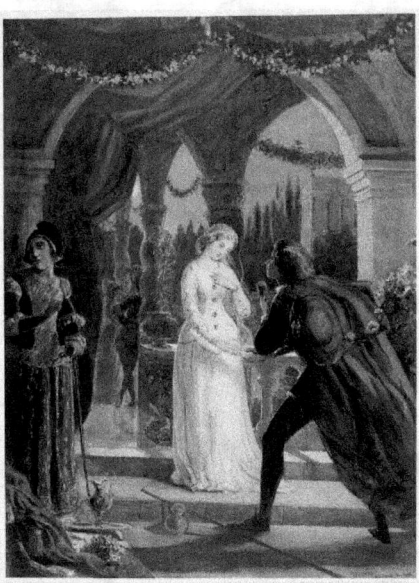

Romeo meets Juliet for the first time.

CHAPTER THREE

RESPONSIBILITY AND PREVENTION PART I

AVOIDING PITFALLS

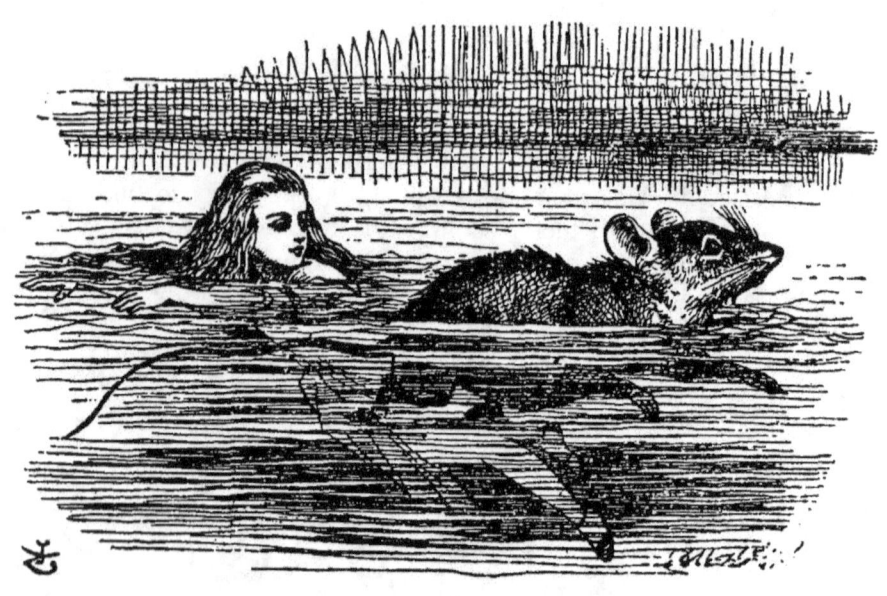

...she soon made out that she was in the pool of tears which she had wept when she was nine feet high. "I wish I hadn't cried so much!" said Alice, as she swam about, trying to find her way out. "I shall be punished for it now, I suppose, by being drowned in my own tears!" Quote from *Alice in Wonderland.*

Interrogate with Interest:

Determine which of these statements are true, and which are false.

1) If a guy asks a girl out, that means they're automatically going steady; seeing anyone else is cheating.

2) Emotionally abusive people are easy to spot, since their behavior is usually obvious.

3) The best time to meet each other's parents is before the first date.

4) Having sex and dabbling in alcohol and drugs are common rites of passage for teens, and is therefore harmless.

5) If you fall for your best friend's date, you should go for it, since all is fair in love and war.

6) Healthy and wholesome living can help a girl avoid date rape.

7) Sticking to environments where people respect each other can help a guy avoid getting raped.

8) A guy will not be harmed by having an affair with an older woman, since guys don't get pregnant.

9) Guys can be just as afraid of sex as girls.

10) Though homophobia exists, there are venues where gays and lesbians can meet each other in a healthy and wholesome atmosphere.

Answers: 1, 2, 4, 5 and 8 are false;
3, 6, 7, 9 and 10 are true.

Dating is a greatly enjoyable experience (or should be, anyway; if it isn't, you're definitely doing something wrong). Its purpose is to discover what sort of person you like, and ultimately, to find a marriage partner. Once you decide to go steady with one particular person, this is your time to get to know one another better.

Many teens – and adults, for that matter – immediately go steady on the first date. It's as if they assume they belong to each other, just because they went out one time. This serious mistake can lead to uncomfortable situations, such as embarrassment if it turns out one partner is not as interested as the other. Also, people who do that often tend to be extremely jealous or possessive, which are signs of an abuser. It is best to date several people at once; ideally, it should start off in groups, so you can get to know lots of kids on a casual basis before going off alone with someone. The first time you go on a solo date, the two of you should meet each other's parents, so they can assess your characters (there are many more reasons; I'll go over them later). After having gone out with one person half a dozen times, then the decision to see each other exclusively should be mutually decided.

Mainly, you will be able to spot and avoid an emotionally abusive partner. Signs are someone who is manipulative; they may use "icing out" and sulking to get what they want. A guy may pressure his girlfriend into having sex early in the relationship, threatening to dump her and ruin her chances of any more dates if she refuses. Or a girl may erode her boyfriend's self-esteem by putting down his achievements and making fun of his goals. The person may be controlling or domineering, constantly demanding you tell them where you are and what you're doing. They may accuse you of things you didn't do, like cheat on them, or blame you for factors beyond your control, like their poor behavior ("I reacted this way because you made me mad"). They may have the habit of co-dependence, which is intruding on someone else's personal boundaries and treating them as an extension of themselves (this is very common among addicts). The aforementioned traits of jealousy and possessiveness are definite giveaways. If you encounter someone like this, *RUN*. It is not your job to "fix" anyone; they need professional help for their problem, which is beyond the scope of practice for high school students. Besides, the only person you can fix is yourself. If you harbor any of these traits, work on getting rid of them, since like attracts like; the more dysfunctional you are, the more likely you will wind up in such a relationship.

COMMON DATING ISSUES

For beginners, I will address the subject of gifts. When choosing a gift, remember that careful consideration will mean far more to the recipient than the price of the gift. So, really listen when you have conversations; that will enable you to select a gift that will be cherished forever.

First, a rundown of gifts *not* to get your date:

For the guy:

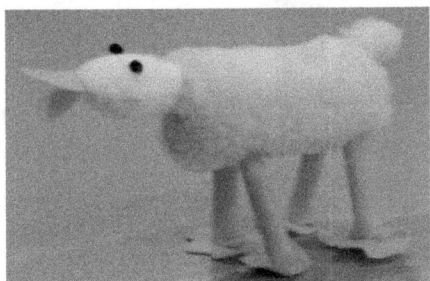

Teenybopper type items. While some girls swoon over stuffed animals and pop idol memorabilia, few guys appreciate them.

For the girl:

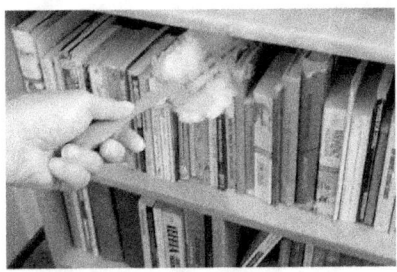

Household cleaning and cooking supplies. On special days, you want to get her mind off the mundane (ironically, it's ok to give a guy a tool kit).

For both:

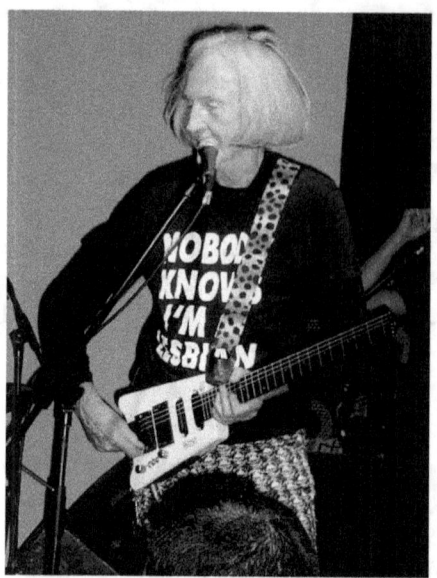

<u>Tacky gifts such as a t-shirt with a sleazy slogan</u>. You want to show you have good taste.

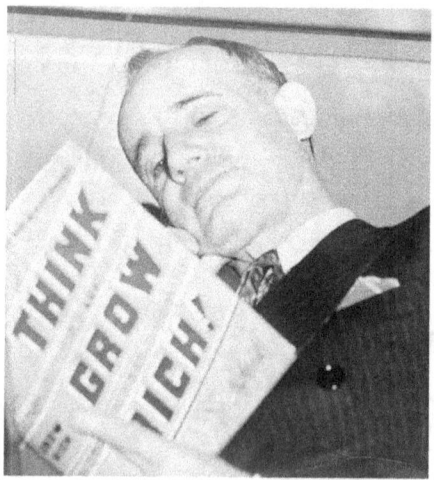

<u>Self-help books</u>. This implies there's something wrong with your partner.

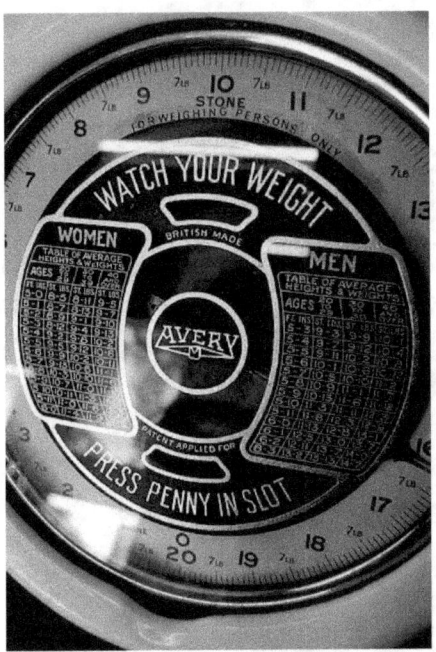

<u>Weight scale</u>. The insult here is obvious.

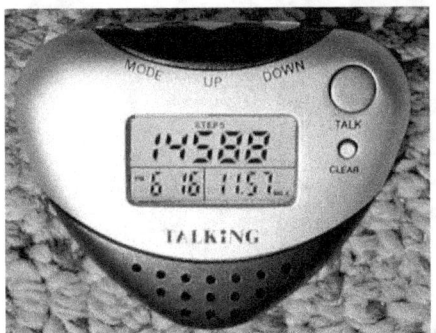

<u>Pedometer.</u> This is almost as insulting as the weight scale.

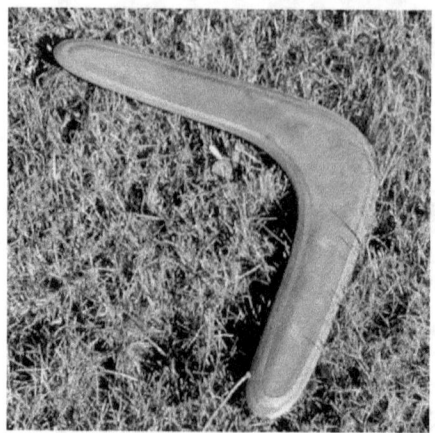

<u>Gift card to *your* favorite store</u>. This is thinly disguised selfishness (the gift boomerangs back to me!).

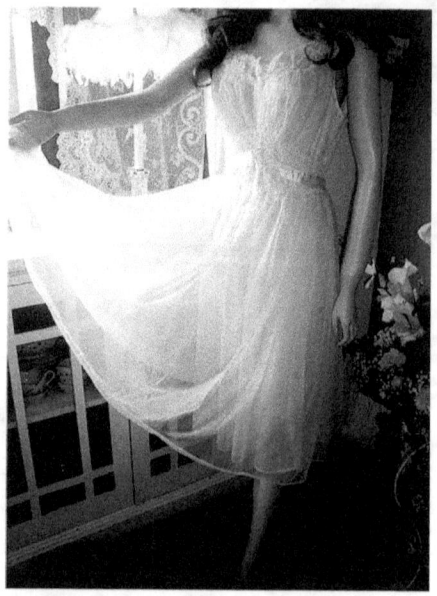

<u>Unless you're both adults – anything of a blatant sexual nature</u>. No sense in leading each other on if you're not of age, or ready for that.

So, what sort of gifts should you get your date? Recordings of their favorite music, t-shirts that commemorate a special event, books, photo albums of shared memories, even basic flowers and chocolates will do. You can buy white flowers and have them dyed in your date's favorite color, for a unique touch.

Good gift ideas for your date

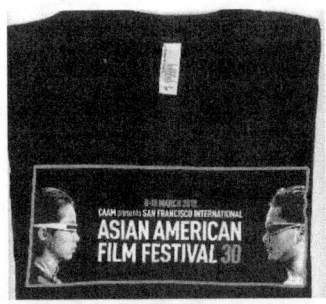
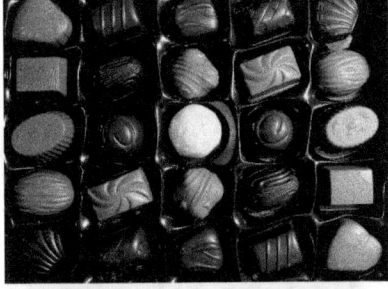
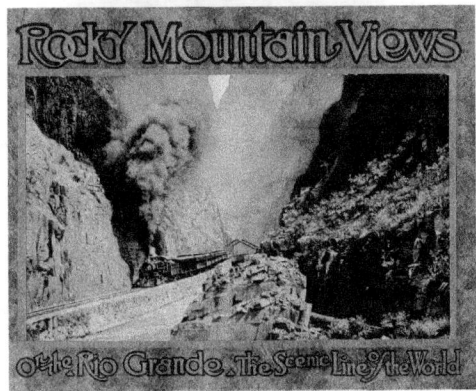
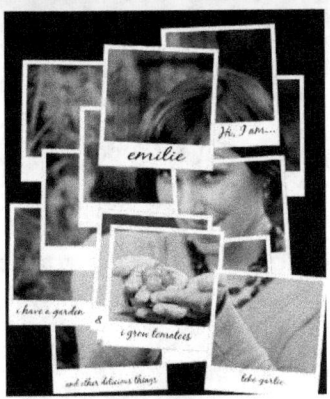
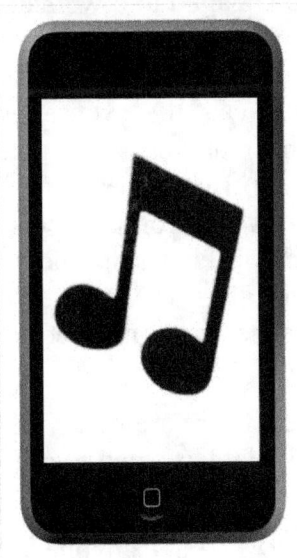
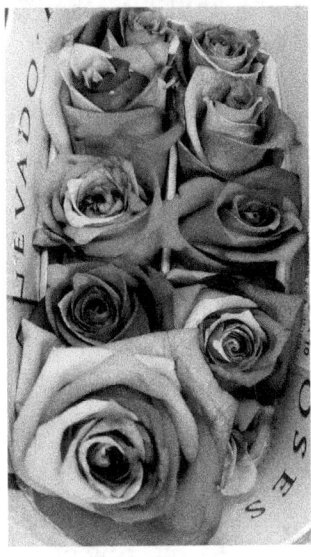

Next, I will address problems that often arise in the dating scene. These scenarios have occurred as long as people have dated, so regardless of how those involved in it feel, it is definitely nothing new.

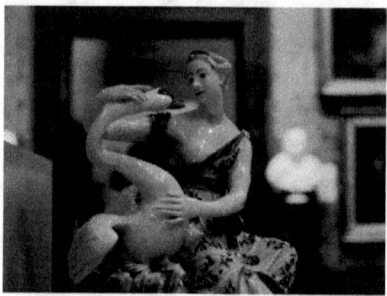

Zeus, disguised as a swan, seduces Leda, Tyndareus' wife.

Stealing someone else's partner. A girl is jealous of her best friend because she is dating a really hot guy, so she tells him lies that cause them to break up so she could get him. Or a guy wants the beauty queen his friend is seeing exclusively, so he does stuff to charm her away from him.

I will first address the thief in this trio. a) How do you know you're going to succeed? If the couple discovers what you're up to, not only will you lose your friend, plus any chance of winning the object of your affection, but also the respect of everyone else who finds out. b) Even if you succeed, what have you gained? Someone who can easily be stolen. How do you know he or she won't be stolen from you? c). Bear in mind the lives of victims have been ruined because of this. I personally know a case where a man who had miraculously kicked heroin became engaged to a woman he was madly in love with, after dating her only a few months. He was immature and inexperienced, and most likely had no business considering marriage yet; no doubt that was the excuse his "best friend" used in stealing her away. The man reacted by fleeing a thousand miles to another city. His "best friend", realizing he may have caused him to relapse, dumped the woman on the spot. I don't know if the jilted lover went back on heroin, but I do know he was murdered several months later. As for the "best friend", I understand guilt consumed him to the point where he never married, even 20 years later.

No one is worth having at that price. There are plenty of people out there who are both desirable and available; expend your energy seeking them.

Next, to the object of affection: *DO NOT* let anyone play this mess on you! As you can tell by the preceding paragraphs, people who do this lack character; most likely, it's only a matter of time before they dump you to run their game on someone else. Also, the relationship you have won't be a real one, since it's based on falsehood, whether it be lying about the other person or charming you through a fake persona. Nobody worth having would do this. If someone says something negative about your girlfriend or boyfriend, investigate the matter rather than assuming it's true. If someone is trying to charm you away, make it clear you're not interested.

Last – but by no means least – I address the victim of this issue. Of course, it's incredibly painful to have someone stolen from you, but ultimately, what have you lost? Someone who can't be trusted. Is someone like that worth having? Even if you manage to win him or her back, it's only a matter of time before it happens again. *PLEASE* do not flip out like the young man I mentioned earlier! Your life has far more value than this. The best way to handle the situation is to make it clear to your partner he or she is free to choose, and you will not cling. Being nice to your rival might throw the person off. Agonizing as it is, free yourself to find someone who will treat you well. Realize you're the better person; after all, it wasn't you that strayed. Maintain your dignity and confidence; if someone throws the incident in your face, calmly state, "Obviously, my ex is a cheater; I can do better than that." Avoid taking revenge; they will bring payback on themselves.

Slut shaming. A guy dates a girl, then spreads false rumors about going all the way. Or a group of girls is jealous of someone who is popular, and scandalizes her reputation, saying the reason guys like her so much is because she sexually puts out all the time. (Guys as a rule are not slut-shamed; instead, they're accused of being gay.)

This is a form of bullying. Kids can have restraining orders placed against them, or even be sued for their future assets, because of this type of behavior. Due to recent

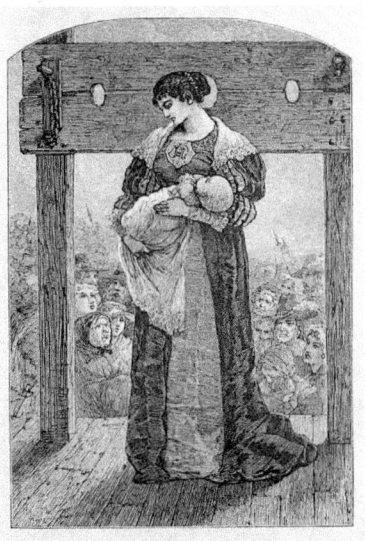

Hester Pyrnne endures scorn in The Scarlet Letter

55

incidents in which victims have been driven to commit suicide, mass murder, or both, schools are beginning to take harassment of all types more seriously, especially since they can be sued as well. Guys and girls who spread malicious rumors should be told flat out that such behavior will not be tolerated; if they continue, avoid associating with them. If you are victimized by said rumors, confront the kids spreading them, saying it's a shame they can't find anything better to do with their lives than sink to this level. Report them to appropriate authorities immediately, and seek counseling to deal with whatever resulting issues you have.

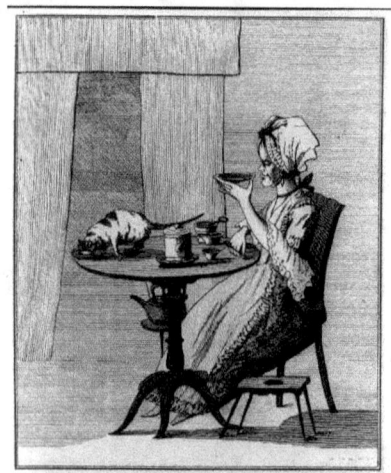

Old Maid

Some people are convinced no one will ever want them, so they cling to anyone who gives them the time of day. This is more common among girls, due to the fact that they're taught to define themselves by their relationships and society judges them more harshly in this category. However, some guys do this too. Often, such people will rush into marriage with no thought regarding what they may be in for. A desperate attitude, which stems from poor self-esteem, is dangerous because abusers often seek out such partners, waiting until they are in a vulnerable spot before launching the exploitation.

A woman from my childhood church was in her mid-20's and, feeling like an undesirable spinster, was anxious to get married. She started dating a wealthy older man who was not a member. He made a great show of being converted and baptized, but once the vows were exchanged, he never set foot in church again. It took eight years of enduring beatings and horrible denigration, aging her and giving her a grayish pallor, before she finally developed the courage to divorce him. Later, she admitted she knew he was like that before the wedding, but was more afraid of ending up an old maid. So she went through all that to gain status that ultimately proved to be worthless.

A young man from this same church attended a faith-based university, met a woman there, and married her 10 months later. I noticed a few days before the wedding, he became quite cranky. When I asked him why, he said it was nerves. I found it strange that his bride didn't display any misgivings whatsoever.

It turned out she was after the Golden Ring Status. She was a horrible housekeeper, rarely cooked, and their two children were raised in an atmosphere of utter chaos, changing schools nearly every year. Much later, the man told me the real reason for his prenuptial bad mood was because he knew she was like that, and had almost called off the wedding. When I asked why he didn't, he said it was because he lacked the courage, and he figured since the two attended a Christian university, God would work things out. In reality, both came from very dysfunctional backgrounds, and had no idea how to conduct a marriage. As it is, he finally divorced her 21 years later, but it was too late to undo the damage.

How can you avoid these situations? Build up your self-esteem by discovering and developing your talents, and working on your shortcomings, whatever they may be. Also, be aware it is a two way street; make an effort to reach out to people and see them as they *truly* are, rather than merely a means to an end. If you're contorting yourself and hiding certain aspects to attract a potential mate, you're missing signs in that other person; being sincere and viewing him or her realistically will save you from being thus deceived. The surest way to avoid such a manipulator is to not be one yourself.

As for people who pass judgement, the best way to deal with them is to give snappy answers to their rude questions. Here are some examples:

<u>"Why don't you have a boyfriend / girlfriend?"</u>

"I'm waiting for your brother / sister to turn 12" (if the boor is an adult, you could say son or daughter).

"Why should I settle for just one?"

"I'd love to be a welfare slut butt / pimp, except that doesn't seem to be working out for me."

"Are you gay?"

"Why? Are you trying to recruit?"

"Why? Are you the alternative?"

"That's not what your mama / daddy thought last night."

Most people who ask such questions have a lot of negativity in their lives, and are putting you down in a vain effort to make themselves feel better. A zesty comeback is the best way to put them in their place. Many of these sarcastic responses came from this link: http://www.ishouldhavesaid.net/ .   You can find many more online, by typing "snappy answers to rude questions" in your search engine.

Obsessing over someone. A girl has a huge crush on a guy; he's unavailable, but she can't get him out of her mind. A guy is stuck over breaking up with his girlfriend. A "popular" person embarrasses his or her date in public, then rubs it in the person's face at every opportunity.

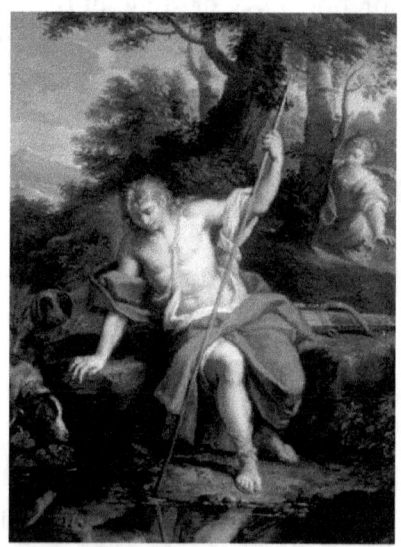

In the first scenario, when you feel yourself attracted to someone, immediately try to make friends with him. Discover his character and interests, what he's truly like, instead of building him up in your fantasies to idol status. If he's unavailable, move on by occupying yourself with other matters. Every-

Echo turns into a mere shadow of herself, obsessing over unavailable Narcissus.

one has their own personal agenda, so there are all sorts of reasons why things don't pan out; you may not be his type, he may be at a time in life when he's not ready, or you two may be incompatible on some other level. Either way, it is best to face facts early; you have partnerships with *real* people, not images. Obsessing over a person you can't get is usually a sign that 1) your life is empty, and you need to fill it with more constructive activities; 2) you're lacking in a certain vital relationship, and you're vainly trying to fill it with a high school kid who can't possibly make up the shortfall; 3) you have a bad habit of always wanting what you can't have. Get counseling to deal with these issues; mentally clinging to someone who is unavailable prevents you from meeting someone who is. If you actually got that person, most likely you would quickly lose interest, or far worse, wind up in Scenario #3 in which he either toys with your emotions or uses you for something far worse. I personally witnessed a girl who was totally enamored over an uninterested guy who proved to be a master manipulator; he enticed her into dropping out of high school to join his cult!

If you wind up in Scenario #3, the best way out is to break yourself off and make it clear to him or her you're no longer interested – or never were in the first place. If the person persists, a little public humiliation may be necessary. Usually, people who run that game show signs early, such as acting overly interested, then being aloof. End contact *THE FIRST TIME* they does this; the longer you continue, the harder it will be to get rid of them.

In Scenario #2, you were already in a relationship, and now it's ending. This extremely painful situation is made worse if you cling to your former partner. Difficult as it is, the best way to handle it is to make a clean break. Tell your former partner that you're glad to have had the experience of a relationship with her, then move on. Keep yourself busy with other activities, so you don't dwell on what used to be. Continuing to cling deprives you of finding someone more suitable, can lead to your former partner manipulating you, and the possibility of being labeled a stalker with ensuing consequences. It will definitely not bring back what you once had, so it's much better to move on to better prospects.

This leads to the complication of how to get out of a partnership. Since middle and high school is a personal era of tremendous change, few relationships last. Couples break up for all sorts of reasons; loss of interest, incompatibility, negative discoveries about the other, need to focus on studies / activities, or just plain weariness of being tied to one person. Before becoming exclusive, it is prudent to know the judicious way out of the situation.

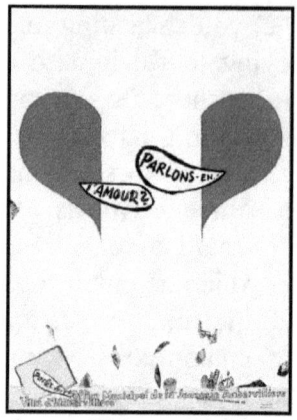

How do you break up with someone? While there is no painless method, you can ease things by being as sensitive and tactful as possible. Start by saying you need to discuss the relationship, then state that you need to break things off because there's no longer any chemistry between you, or to focus on other matters, or see other people. If the other has blatant faults, such as violent temper or messing with drugs or alcohol, specifically say so, but in a way that will benefit him or her. Afterwards, allow your former partner time apart from you. Perhaps you two can remain friends, but accept the fact that it may not happen; if it does, it will take awhile for the other person to recover. Avoid breaking up by lashing out in anger in the middle of an argument, or taking the cowardly route through texting or over the phone. Also, do not do it in public, unless you're in danger of physical retaliation.

HOMOSEXUALITY

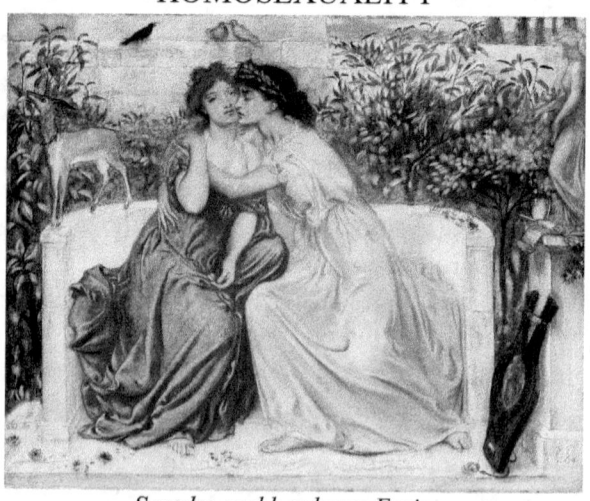

Sappho and her lover Errina,
from the Isle of Lesbos, Greece

The teen years are the time of life when people discover their sexual orientation. Same sex crushes are common among young children, but after puberty, most become attracted to the opposite

60

gender. A few do not; that is when they discover they are homosexual.

It is still not clear what causes homosexuality. In the past, it was believed to be due to the way children were raised, or blamed on emotional trauma at a vulnerable time, but more and more, it is becoming evident that the basis is genetic. Another unknown is how many homosexuals there are. Americans estimate the number to be as high as 20%, with more prevalence among females. However, statistics show it to be less than 4%, with men outnumbering women by nearly 2 to 1.

Homosexuals can have a difficult time meeting potential partners because, unfortunately, homophobia is a major factor in American society. The situation is improving; the Supreme Court has recently even legalized same-sex marriage, but homosexuals still face discrimination in many areas. If you're lucky enough to live in a liberal city, you can join social groups that cater to gays; an example is the Different Spokes Bicycling Club in Seattle. If, on the other hand, your environment is oppressive, contact PFLAG, which stands for Parents and Friends of Lesbians and Gays. Here is a link to their website: http://community.pflag.org/ . They can direct you to local resources, and assist in issues such as coming out to your parents. Once you're on your own, you can relocate to a more accepting location. Once there, check out the local university; most have gay and lesbian groups where people gather and discuss issues, and they can help you find activities to join. Make sure you stick to healthy and wholesome ones; avoid the bar and bathhouse scene, since young people are often taken advantage of there.

HAVING SEX

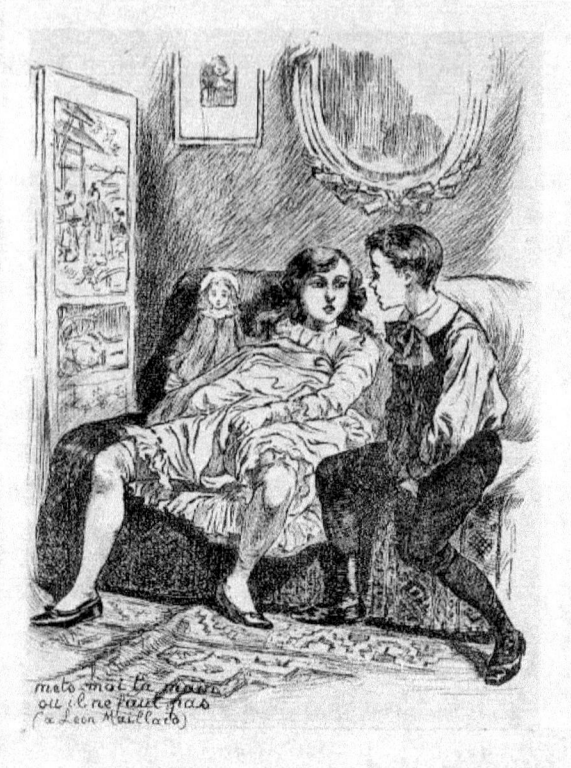

"Put your hand where it's not right."

The general consensus is, "Everybody's doing it". Yet, statistics present an entirely different picture; only about half of high school students have ever had sex, with 17 being the most common age for their first experience.

Listed below are reasons why high school students shouldn't have sex.

1) <u>They usually know very little about it</u>. I once read a story of a teen couple who used to make out all the time. Then one day the girl was home alone, and decided she wanted to lose her virginity. She called her boyfriend to come over, and they finally went all the way. She wondered why it wasn't enjoyable, and was downright painful. There's a lot more involved in sex than the act.

2) <u>They have not considered the consequences.</u> What do you know about STDs? What type of birth control will you use? What if it fails and the girl gets pregnant?

3) <u>They are seldom emotionally mature enough to handle it</u>. Many teens feel squeamish about even discussing the aforementioned topics, so how can they actually deal with it – or the aftermath, if they don't deal with it, or if things go wrong? (Example; a girl can get an abortion, but both parties will be scarred for life due to the gut-wrenching decision of terminating the pregnancy). Sex can also cloud one's judgment; you can feel bonded to the person, making it difficult to leave the relationship after finding out later he or she has undesirable characteristics.

4) <u>What are the Age of Consent laws in your state</u>? Not knowing can get you into BIG trouble. There are instances where guys have been listed as sex offenders because they had sex with their girlfriends who were slightly under 18!

5) <u>Succumbing to peer pressure is one of the worst reasons for having sex.</u> Especially if you don't really know what your peers are doing. Also, the crowd that is having sex may very well be the loser crowd.

6) <u>An emotionally immature person may have sex to try to win someone's love, or be "grown up".</u> The former is manipulative, the latter foolish. Manipulation repels desirable people and attracts dysfunctional ones; rather than love you, the person will most likely use you. Likewise, you prove your adulthood by being responsible, not screwing around.

The time to have sex is when you're of age, know your partner well (this takes *AT LEAST* six months of seeing each other exclusively, with *LOTS* of open communication; some believe you should wait until after marriage), and both of you have fully educated yourselves on the subject, including birth control and STD prevention. No pressures, secrecy or control issues should be involved in the decision-making process. The two of you need to discuss whatever consequences might come up, and how you will deal with them. Contrary to popular belief, declining sex is not that tricky, and you don't need a million ways to do it. Just avoid situations which will tempt you, like being alone together in isolated places, and politely tell your partner you're not ready yet; you need to know each other better, develop emotionally, and be prepared to deal with whatever may come up. Anyone worth having will respect this; if they don't, you're better off without them.

Why do guys push their girlfriends into having sex? Many times they believe that's what they really want, but it can turn out to be more than they bargained for. Peer pressure plays a part, or proving their "manhood". Or it could be simply to show they're interested. I once heard a story about a man who propositioned a woman on the third date, and when she declined, he actually thanked her. He told her he wasn't ready for sex either; he just wanted to show her he cared.

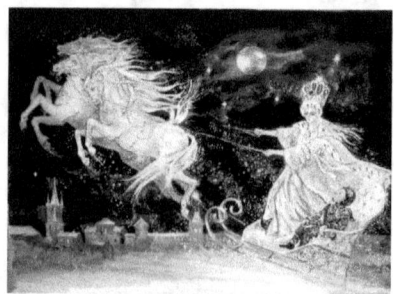

The evil Snow Queen runs off with Kai, Gerda's childhood sweetheart.

Here, I need to add a note for high school guys. No doubt you have heard of recent cases in the news about female teachers having affairs with male students, some as young as 12 years old. You may think this is a desirable situation, and boys can escape it unscathed, but that is *NOT TRUE*. This is child molestation, no different from if the genders were reversed. Being used as a sex object wreaks havoc on a boy's emotional development; going from zero to ten in nothing flat prevents them from learning how to court girls and manage the nuances of a relationship. Inevitably, they later resent being used, with some going on to become child molesters or rapists. Also, a boy can impregnate a woman, who then turns around and sues him or his parents for child support. Imagine having to be financially responsible for a baby on a part-time minimum wage job, before you've saved up for your first car! And it will go on for *EIGHTEEN YEARS!*

Women who seek out boys for sexual relationships are usually extremely immature and on a power trip. There is a story on the web about a 12-year-old boy who had an affair with a baby sitter, already divorced at the ripe old age of 22. She used to make him vow to marry her soon as he was old enough – this, when he'd never even had a girlfriend. Later, when he was 17, he had a brief affair with a woman who had separated from her husband. It turned out she was using him too; when she decided to give her marriage another try, she dumped him on the spot. Fortunately, he later met a wonderful girl his age who was able to help him work through the resulting emotional wreckage, and they are still married after 30 – odd years. However, many are not so lucky. Regarding the news cases, follow what happens to the boys involved, and find out what becomes of them.

As you can see, such women make lousy partners anyway. Never approach an adult for sex, no matter how attractive you find her. Likewise, if she approaches you, *REFUSE*. If she harasses you, report her to your parents, or a minister or counselor, so they can deal with the situation. You will have plenty of opportunities in your lifetime to find someone who is both desirable and appropriate.

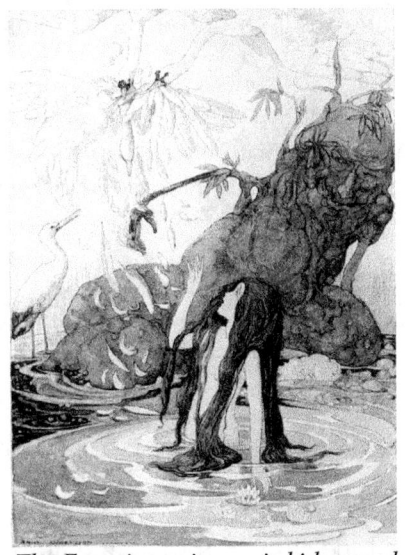

The Egyptian princess is kidnapped by the vile Marsh King.

Likewise, girls should stay strictly away from men who want to "school" them. The dangers in such situations are well-known; it is a surefire way to become a crime victim. Many times these monsters are recruiting streetwalkers, the lowest form of prostitution and currently the most common form of human trafficking. At the very least, as soon as he gets you pregnant, he'll abandon you, leaving you to face decisions that will adversely affect your life forever.

DATE RAPE

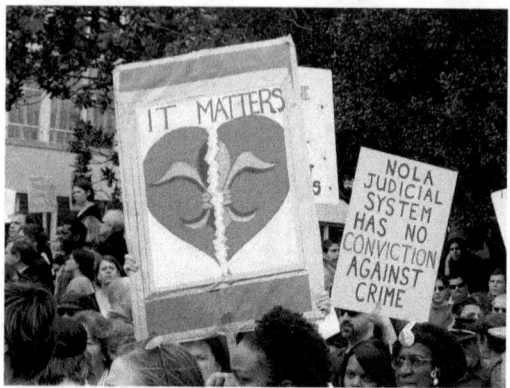

It breaks the law as well as the heart.

Date rape is using physical force or emotional coercion to get sex on a date. A guy can commit this act without realizing what he is doing, so he needs to learn that a no means *NO*. He can serve sentence for not respecting boundaries. I know a case where a guy wrestled with a girl in a grocery store. He was most likely just being stupid and immature, since rapists know better than to commit the act in public places, but the girl reported him, and he wound up spending 30 days in jail. He will be registered as a sex offender the rest of his life, prohibiting him from working in certain job fields. All this before he turned 18!

How can a girl avoid date rape? Having the guy meet her parents before the first date is an excellent idea; while most guys aren't rapists, this should intimidate one who would think of doing such a thing. Also, meeting his parents gives her an idea of what sort of home he comes from, giving perspective to his character. If they were involved in the same social group at school, that should give her insight from the start.

Other ways to avoid date rape are:

1) <u>Do not drink or use drugs, and refuse to attend parties where people do this</u>. Alcohol and drugs negatively affect judgment, and render you less able to fight off an attacker. Date rape drugs can be slipped into an alcoholic drink (non-alcoholic, in some instances) while the person isn't looking, making them unconscious and remembering nothing when they sober up. The crime can

be difficult to report since you may not even know who raped you. To make matters worse, while unconscious, victims have been defiled and photographed and their pictures posted on the web. There are plenty of ways to have a good time that don't involve fogging your brain; stick to those.

2) Trust your instincts. If anyone makes you feel uncomfortable, don't go off alone with him. Sometimes rapists put out a vibe of being a total loser that thinks nothing of taking advantage of someone. I once had a girlfriend who rarely went out. When she finally got a date, she proudly introduced me and some others to him. I picked up on that vibe. Unfortunately, at the time I didn't know what it meant; I just assumed he was as desperate for a date as she was (if I had known, I definitely would have pulled her aside and warned her!). The next day, she told us he had driven them to an isolated spot and tried to rape her; she was lucky to be able to jump out of the car and run to safety. What became of the case is another story; however, several years later, I was watching a newscast where three rapists were being interviewed, and I felt that same vibe coming from the screen (it would be a good idea for you to look up such an interview on YouTube, to get an idea). Rape is not an act of passion; it is a form of bullying that simply takes on a sexual nature. Not all bullies are rapists, but all rapists are bullies.

3) Date only guys who respect girls. Have nothing to do with someone who despises them, or sees them as lesser people. If you harbor such attitudes towards guys, get counseling to change that before dating, since like attracts like.

4) In addition, avoid guys – and girls – who don't respect you. I'm talking about people who accuse you of being "hypersensitive" when you call them on inappropriate behavior, or being uptight if you refuse to do something against your values. Also, beware of those with violent,

hair-trigger tempers. While this does not always lead to date rape, it signifies an abusive relationship. One reason women become battered wives is because of the company they keep; I have been told by several that over half the women they know are beaten on a regular basis, even though the national average is closer to thirty percent for a single incident.

5) <u>Wait until you know each other well before going off alone</u>. Hanging out in the same group and meeting each other's family helps towards that end.

6) <u>Make your intentions clear regarding sex</u>. Make up your mind beforehand how far to go, and stick to it. Guys; no means *NO!* (Refer to the grocery store incident I told above, to see what could happen if you disregard this.)

7) <u>Take self-defense courses, so you're better able to protect yourself if a problem comes up</u>. You may also want to carry pepper spray; check the laws in your state (here's a link: <u>http://www.misdefenseproducts.com/Pepper-Spray-Laws-Restrictions-sp-6.html</u>). Make sure you're trained how to use, and keep it within easy reach.

Incidentally, guys get raped too. It usually happens when they're in a "rape culture" setting, such as a prison, or any rough crowd that bullies, blames victims, and basically disregards human rights. While less common, it can be even more devastating, because of the stigma involved. It is assumed guys are invincible to that sort of thing, or that they always want sex so the victim must be homosexual and therefore asked for it (the fact that homophobia is alive and well in this country makes matters worse). However, it is *EXTREMELY* important that anyone with this unfortunate experience report it immediately. Go to the hospital and demand a rape kit, even if you were only mildly injured. See a qualified counselor as soon as possible; you can even chat anonymously through the Rape Abuse & Incest National Network (RAINN) website (<u>https://www.rainn.org/</u>). Rapists often attack dozens of people before they're caught, so you'll be protecting future potential victims as well.

ALCOHOL AND DRUGS

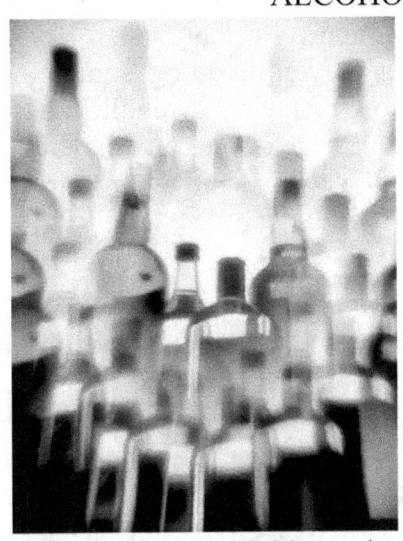

The drinking age is 21 all over the US, for good reason; the brain continues to grow and develop until age 25, so introducing alcohol too early can stunt its growth. College campuses have had a huge problem with drunkenness, so in 1987 the national age limit was raised to 21, above that of the average student (though it still continues to be a problem; by the way, most campus rapes happen at keg parties). Studies have shown the earlier someone starts drinking, the more likely they will become an alcoholic, the faster it will happen, and the harder the addiction will be to overcome.

Perhaps you're wondering 1) should people drink at all? or 2) many countries in Europe don't even have a drinking age, so what's the big deal? Here's the answer to both: alcoholism is largely determined by psychology and culture. If an adult *makes the decision* to drink excessively every day, it takes years for physical addiction and loss of control to sneak up on him or her; months if the drinker is under age 15. Bad habits like binge drinking (consuming large amounts in one session, which is common among underage drinkers), hiding and lying about how much you drink, behaving irresponsibly while drinking (like driving under the influence rather than timing yourself or getting a designated driver beforehand), and drinking to relieve stress or escape a bad mood can lead to the cumulative effect of addiction. In other words, it is a form of choice. In Europe, children learn early how to consume alcohol responsibly, and drunkenness is frowned upon. Some countries have extremely harsh drunk driving laws; in Sweden, it is 10 years of hard labor for the first offense! On the other hand, in the Americas alcohol is often seen as "forbidden fruit", and people are less likely to be taught responsibility regarding its consumption. As a result, though Europe has the most drinkers, North and South America have the most alcoholics. Alcohol is to be used for pleasant socializing by mature people who will be responsible with it, and for celebrations. If you have to be deceitful about your usage, you're doing something wrong. Obviously, no one sets out to become an alcoholic, so of course you'll say you won't choose to become one, but if you're strong enough to deal with it and not get hooked, you're strong enough to wait until you're 21; then you'll have the rest of your life to enjoy it without guilt or fear.

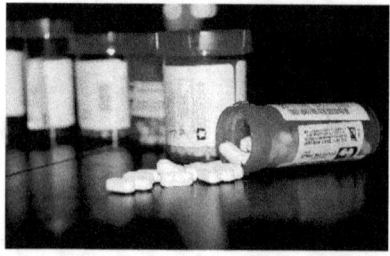

A recent trend is the abuse of prescription and over-the-counter medications. These serve specific purposes; to relieve pain, induce sleep, ease cold and flu symptoms, suppress appetite, alleviate depression, treat ADHD, or increase energy. Taken as the doctor ordered or in the dosages indicated on the package, they are relatively harmless. However, mixing with other meds, taking them in too large amounts, or using for reasons other than what they were meant, can do damage, some of it irreversible. It can cause poisoning that result in a coma, seizures, paralysis, even death. Medication abuse may also wear out the nerve receptors to the point where they no longer serve their purpose. I've known a couple of people who can no longer get pain relief, even with the strongest antidotes. One woman was in the hospital for surgery; even Demerol shots couldn't help her, and she spent three days in agony, unable to sleep because of it.

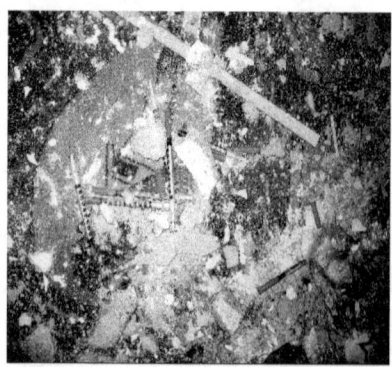

As for illegal drugs, the highly addictive ones are currently used as shackles for sex trade human trafficking. Often a "cool" adult appearing to love a good time (but in reality is a recruiting pimp and drug dealer) will hold parties and invite teens – guys as well as girls – over to try all they want for free. Some, like meth, can hook a person the first time they use. Others, like heroin, may take as long as 2 weeks. Either way, once they're hooked, it's usually for life, and then they're forced to become streetwalkers to support their habits, making the pimp / drug dealer rich in the process. If they run away, they go through life-threatening withdrawals. To kick the drugs, they need medical assistance, which the pimp isn't about to provide. Even with the ones lucky enough to escape and go through rehab, success is rare. You may say, "Well, smoking weed isn't going to do this", but marijuana, alcohol, even cigarettes, are gateway drugs. You try those, get bored with them, and then are tempted to move on to something stronger, and you lie to yourself, thinking it won't hook you if you use only every once in a while. But that's what *ALL* addicts say. Remember, no one deliberately sets out to get hooked. Keep this in mind, when someone tries to temp you to use. True, not all addicts wind up as victims of human trafficking, but it definitely makes them more vulnerable (I know of a situation where a college football / basketball player dabbled in crack for years, but ultimately wound up being forced to support his habit by disguising himself as a woman and working as a streetwalker). In all cases it ruins health, looks, and quality of life. You can find *LOADS* of ways to have fun without going that route, and you'll thank yourself later when you're older and wiser (your future spouse and children will thank you too!).

EROTICA / PORNOGRAPHY

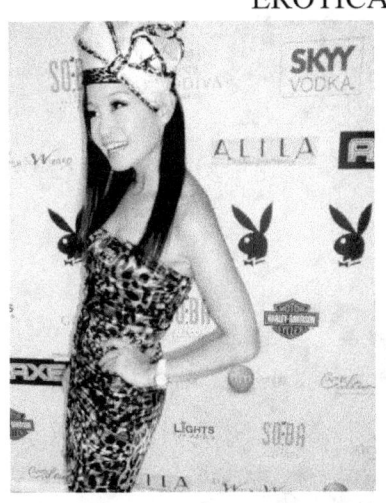 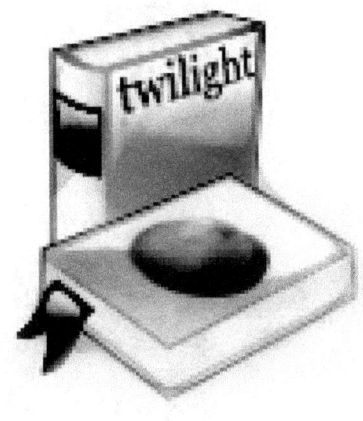

I will end the chapter with this subject. When people don't have access to sex on a regular basis, they often use erotica to let off steam. Since guys are turned on by sight, they enjoy looking at sexy images of nude women; meanwhile, girls, who are turned on by situations, prefer reading confession magazines. As long as this doesn't affect your outside relationships or expectations, it is harmless. When it interferes with your life to the point of addiction (the rate is 17%, double that of alcoholism), it is time to get help from a counselor. Just a few words of caution; avoid online porn, since several sites contain viruses. Also, you must be 18 to view an X-rated movie, and many are made under unethical conditions, so if you go that route, first check out what the actors have to say about working conditions on social media.

This is a lot of information to take in, but it is important. Study it often, committing it to memory. As the saying goes, forewarned is forearmed!

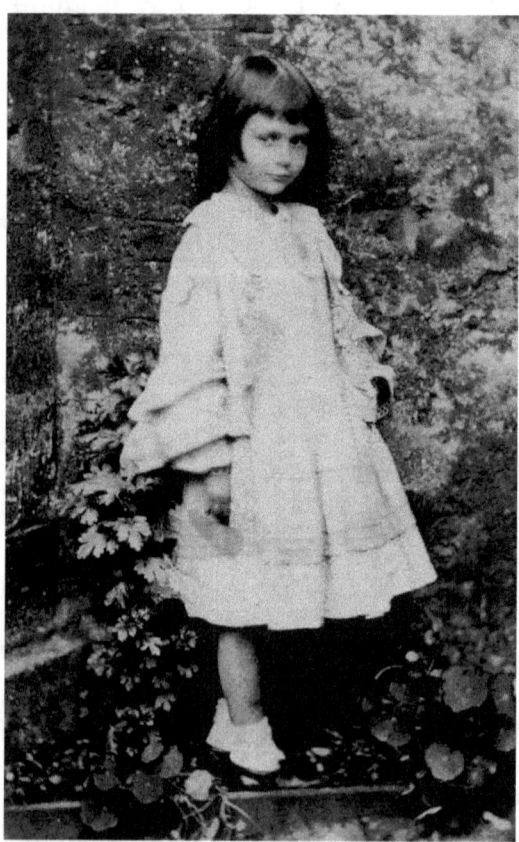

The real Alice in Wonderland

Toil over the Turmoil:

1) You live in an area that is rife with drugs. Write a list of ways you and your friends can live a healthy and wholesome lifestyle and engage in activities without drugs. Hint: sports and drugs don't mix!

2) Where you live, disrespect for the opposite sex is rampant. Rap music, movie portrayals, reality TV and lewd music videos exacerbate the issue. Discuss this with your friends, parents, and teachers of both genders. While discussing, compare the social scene of today with the way it was 50 - 100 years ago. Include all ethnicities (special note: Dick Gregory, African American comedian, grew up in St. Louis during the 1930s and 1940s; his was the only family in the neighborhood headed by a single mother). Do research on the internet, if necessary. In the past, people had to treat each other better because they needed each other. Though technology has rendered this less necessary, what would happen to society if it continues on this path?

3) You live in an area where violence is rampant. Discuss ways with your teachers and parents that young people can enjoy activities without being victimized, or being forced to join a gang for safety. Hint: there is safety in numbers!

CHAPTER FOUR

RESPONSIBITLY AND PREVENTION PART II

THE COMPANY YOU KEEP – REAL AND VIRTUAL

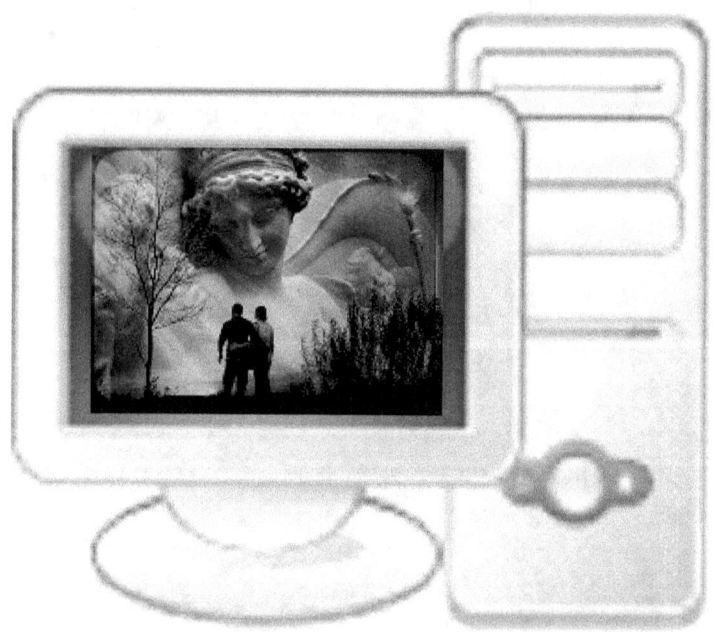

Who is looking out for you?

Inversion

Determine which of these statements are true, and which are false.

1) The internet has made the world one giant neighborhood. Because of it, you can now be friends with someone with whom you don't share a common language.

2) Being harassed over the internet (cyberbullying) is no big deal, since it is not done in person and can't result in physical harm.

3) Internet social groups protect users from predators, since no one can be harmed unless they meet in person.

4) The best way to deal with internet trolls (troublemakers) is to refuse to give them the attention they crave.

5) When making purchases over the internet, or placing an order by phone, it is best to pay by credit card.

6) When a pop-up screen tells you to click on it for an update, it is safe for you to do so.

7) All cults are based on religion.

8) The internet is ideal for spreading cults and hate groups worldwide.

9) Though all religions have cult offshoots, some have more than others.

10) People who belong to a religion that has Absolute Truth are least likely to cults.

Answers: 2, 3, 6, 7 and 10 are false;
1, 4, 5, 8 and 9 are true.

arlier in this book, I have mentioned several times that people should meet each other's parents before going on the first date, listing the reasons to do so. Unfortunately, that is not feasible for kids from abusive homes, or for adults who have moved far from their families or whose parents are deceased. In this case, a person's social circle can serve the purpose of screening dates and testifying to the person's character. Some excellent resources are Boys and Girls Clubs of America, Girl Scouts and Boy Scouts, and volunteer associations run by the Kiwanis. You can also look into sports and arts leagues led by your school and church. Some people find social networking difficult, but the more good friends one has, the greater his or her advantages; through them, you can learn positive ways of relating, and make connections for getting good jobs in the future. Likewise, check out your potential date's social group; that tells you something about them.

This is a good time to bring up the subject of internet communities. Social sites enable you to interact with people all over the world; you can become best friends with someone you've never met and, using Google Translate, with whom you may not even share a common language! While the internet has done much to make the world one big neighborhood, it also presents unique dangers. You can be harassed and bullied by anonymous people, making it difficult to defend yourself while being publicly humiliated; you can be financially robbed and have your identity stolen, possibly being arrested for crimes you didn't commit; you can even be assaulted or kidnapped if you meet an online "friend" in person, only to discover they are nothing like their profile. Because it is so difficult to legally regulate the internet, detrimental sites abound. Some sell stolen goods, promote false get-rich-quick schemes, or teach how to create fake IDs, forge counterfeit money, manufacture bombs and produce illegal drugs. Not only may you get involved with some highly undesirable characters, you can get nabbed by the FBI for visiting such websites. Some can even lure you into getting caught up in child pornography. Then there are those that appear to be convincingly legitimate, but are fronts to garner sensitive information for identity theft.

These are the reasons caring parents establish filters on their children's computers and monitor their use. If you don't have such a screening device, or your parents are technophobes, here are steps you can take to protect yourself (these safety tips apply to adults as well).

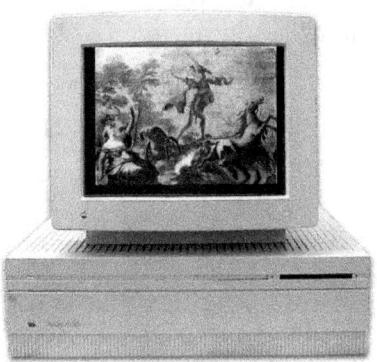

Hades kidnaps Persephone

1) Never disclose personal information on a social site that will enable a stranger to find you. This includes your home address, school, phone number, or place of work. Do not display photos of these locations, either.

2) Be careful what pictures of yourself you post online. Some kids may think it's cool to post themselves partying, but that can backfire if they apply for a job and their future boss comes across those degrading – or incriminating – photos. Remember, everything you put online - words as well as pictures - is available for the whole world to see. In fact, it is best to clear with your parents before you post. *ABSOLUTELY NO NUDIES* – this is child pornography!

3) *NEVER* meet someone in person alone that you first interacted with online! Always bring a parent or trusted adult with you!

4) Check with your parents and / or an internet savvy person before downloading any software. You never know what viruses it may contain.

5) Do not share your password with anyone except your parents. This will save you from being falsely and unfavorably impersonated. It is also a good idea to passcode lock the screen of your computer, laptop and tablet so they cannot be used if stolen. Putting your contact information on the screen may facilitate your equipment being returned to you.

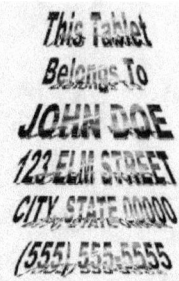

6) You may want to teach your parents what you know about the internet, so they will become comfortable with it.

Following are ways to avoid cyberbullying:

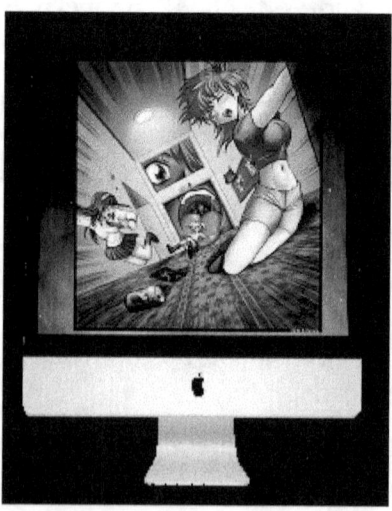

1) Do not respond to cruel messages. If they're on your wall, copy them to a word document, then delete such posts. If they're in a private email, save them, but do not indicate in any way that you're affected by it. (The

reason for saving the offending comments is so you can file a harassment report.) If you're in a chat room and someone comes in hurling insults, the action to take is for everyone to switch to a totally boring topic, like planting trees or the weather in the Sahara Desert. The best way to get rid of trolls (people who cause dissent over the web) is to *NOT FEED THEM*. Avoid friending anyone who makes a habit of stirring up trouble. Likewise, never post anything inappropriate about anyone, whether it be words or pictures. The rule "like attracts like" applies on the internet as well as in real life.

2) Only post online a statement you would say to someone's face. Do not backstab. Better yet, avoid posting negative comments about anyone altogether; discuss the matter in person instead.

3) Depending on the social climate in your area, you may want to use the privacy settings on social websites.

4) If someone makes you uncomfortable, refuse to interact with them. If they harass or cyberstalk you, report the offender to website authorities.

5) Regularly look up your name, to be sure no one has set up false sites using you. Be sure to include common misspellings of your name, since imposters sometimes use that to make it more difficult for them to get caught. If you find a false site, report it to the web host, to Google, and all major search engines, so they can take it down and prosecute the culprit. Depending on state laws and the type / extent of damage, false impersonation online can be a felony.

And now, a list of precautions to take to avoid becoming a cyberspace robbery victim. Scams to get money from unsuspecting users proliferate; a fortune is being offered to you by a wealthy "friend", deceased "relative", or even a generous stranger from a foreign country. They ask you to send them money to assist with taxes, or to bribe officials. Or someone emails you, impersonating someone you know, saying he or she was mugged on vacation and needs your financial help. A very common one is that you won a sweepstakes, and all that is necessary to claim your prize is to send cash using a Green Dot card to cover the small processing fee. Some scammers set up a false site that imitates a charity, asking for donations through it. Most frightening of all are pop-up ads saying your computer is infected, and you need to click on it and pay $50 to buy software to clean it up. If you click on the ad and pay the money, not only is your computer not cleaned, but spyware is downloaded onto it, causing a *real* problem.

Here I will describe the most commons scams. Many of them are geared towards grownups, but swindlers have no qualms against using children to hook their parents. These are the ways both youth and adults can protect themselves against such fraud:

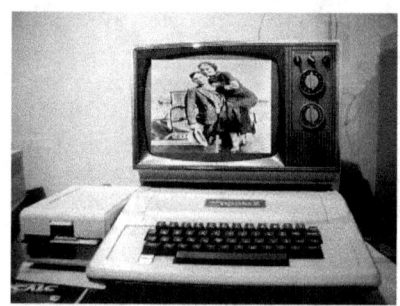

"Trust us – we'll give you an upgrade!"
~ Bonnie & Clyde

1) First off, never send money using wire transfer, money order, pre-loaded card, international funds transfer, electronic currency, Green Dot or debit card, to someone you don't know. Money sent in this manner is rarely recovered; it is easier to retrieve if a credit card was used. Automatically suspect anyone who demands you to pay by any method other than credit card.

2) If a friend wanted to share a fortune with you, they'd tell you in person, wouldn't they? What are the chances of a long-lost relative looking you up? Verify with an independent lawyer to check if you actually have wealthy deceased relatives in Nigeria or some other foreign country. If you find a gorgeous date online, automatically be suspicious if he or she asks for money (one of many good reasons high school kids should not

do internet dating). Sometimes, you may get an actual phone call from a "friend" who has been mugged. In this case, ask the person a question only your friend would know, such as what the two of you did the last time you were together, what they wore, etc. You may want to get on another phone and call your friend at home, to see if they really are in the location where the imposter says they are.

3) If you didn't enter sweepstakes, you didn't win anything. Do not let anyone convince you otherwise! Also, if they're generous enough to give you a couple million dollars, surely they can cover a $500 processing fee. Or they can let you pay them after you get that couple million dollars. (When the telemarketer asked if I had $500, I answered no, but I would after I got that $2 million. He sputtered, then I told him I knew he was a scammer and I was going to report him. He got angry and said I could kiss his @$$! LOL!)

P.S. When I reported him, I was informed there's nothing they can do because those telemarketers call from the (876) area code, which is in Jamaica, outside US jurisdiction. Do not dial such a number; the toll charges are huge! No doubt that's why the guy got angry, because I made him run up a bill giving his spiel, while I knew all along he was a crook.

Update; it is now possible for scamming telemarketers outside the country to obtain a U.S. area code, so don't be fooled if that's what comes up on your phone.

4) A more low-key – and possibly more deceitful – version of this scam is one where you're told you were chosen to receive a package of coupons that can be used at any major store, such as Target or Walmart. All you have to do is send $8 to claim it. You can easily pick up coupons to those stores anywhere for free, so don't fall for it!

5) A frightening scam is a phone call, allegedly from the IRS, threatening to sue for back taxes. This may come as

81

a computerized message, or from an actual person who speaks in an intimidating way. The person may even have the last 4 digits of your social security number. Do not believe them! The IRS does not sue people; if you actually do owe back taxes, they will contact you by mail. They are quite reasonable in helping you work out a deal; at worst, they may garnish up to half your wages, but only if you refuse to cooperate. The IRS never contacts by phone or email. You may want to report the phone call to their website.

6) Anytime someone wants to give you a check, even if it's a cashier's check, for an amount that's larger than an item you're selling, asking you to send them the difference, do not do it! The check is fake. You will lose your real money in the process. A recent scam is a large company having their ad painted on your car, sending you a check to cover the cost of the paint job plus an extra amount you can keep for yourself as payment for advertising. Actually, it is an imposter posing as a representative for that large company; when the check bounces, you're liable for the paint job.

7) Some rental listings ask the potential client to wire them a deposit. After the money is sent, it turns out there is no rental. Always visit the place yourself (that way, you can see if you really want to rent it), and pay the deposit in person.

8) Be *VERY* careful about clicking on certain links! Some scammers send emails from your bank, or various accounts like Amazon, PayPal, or eBay, saying there's a problem with your account, and you need to click on that link to fix it. Clicking on it will take you to a fake site; logging in will enable them to acquire sensitive information, like your password and bank account numbers. If you receive such an email, contact the company, either by phone or by going to your web browser and typing the actual address yourself. Banks and companies do not send emails or phone calls asking

for login or sensitive information, so anyone who does should be suspected.

9) You may get a pre-approved credit card offer by email, saying they will send it to you as soon as you pay the annual fee. Once you pay the fee, you'll never hear from them again. Just say no! Also, you may get an email – or phone call – offering to lower your credit card interest rates, but then they ask you to "verify" your account number. If the company was legitimate, they would already have that information. Pass on it!

10) Another version of this scam is a phone call to renew the warranty on your car. The caller will ask you for its year, make and model, to certify they have the right person. In reality, an extended warranty may not be necessary, either because your car may still be under the original contract, or it may be an excellent car that rarely needs repairs. If you want to buy an extended warranty, you need to research the company to make sure it has a solid reputation, that it actually pays its claims and won't go bankrupt. You also need to determine what type of warranty you need, and to buy it at the correct time – not too soon or too late. Obviously you can't do that over the phone with a telemarketer, so it is definitely a scam. I responded to such a call by telling him I drove a late model Peugeot, and he hung up on me. LOL!

11) Another scam is an offer for a work-at-home job, if you buy something like a website or processing equipment, or a list of contacts. Once you send the money, no job materializes. Oftentimes, neither does the equipment.

12) Rather than respond to emails from charities, visit those sites yourself to make donations. Make sure the charities themselves are legitimate, by checking with the Better Business Bureau.

13) Do not pirate software, music, movies, games or anything. Not only is this unethical (would you want someone to steal the product of your hard work?), people

who deal in such matters are often unscrupulous, thinking nothing of taking advantage of you. Sites that promote piracy often contain viruses; they can steal your identity and damage your computer to the point where you may have to replace it. Always buy your software from a reputable company.

14) People who are overwhelmed with debt should go to the local non-profit Credit Counseling Service. They can help them make deals with their creditors, charging little or nothing for the service. Do not pay someone who offers to wipe out your debt! Only bankruptcy can do that, in which case you need a lawyer. During times of economic crisis, this scam abounds, so be very careful!

15) The internet – and magazines and TV as well – are rife with ads promoting instant cures and weight loss products. They put pressure on the buyer to "act now", because it's only available for a "limited time". Obviously, any product that can make a person lose 50 pounds in 5 days or cure cancer would fly off the shelves, so why do they offer it only for a limited time? Don't waste your money! Instead, go to your doctor and discuss any issues you have.

16) Regarding the "infection detected" pop-up ads – install a legitimate spyware program on your computer immediately after getting it. If you get such a pop-up ad, shut down your computer without closing any windows, either using control-alt-delete or pressing the power button, and reboot it. If that doesn't solve the problem, look for the rogue program in your task manager and delete it. If that still doesn't solve the problem, take your computer to a professional.

The internet is a fabulous place to interact, learn, and expand your horizons – if used wisely. However, be careful not to become addicted. Remember your real time friends - they're the most important!

POLITICS VERSUS PROPOGANDA

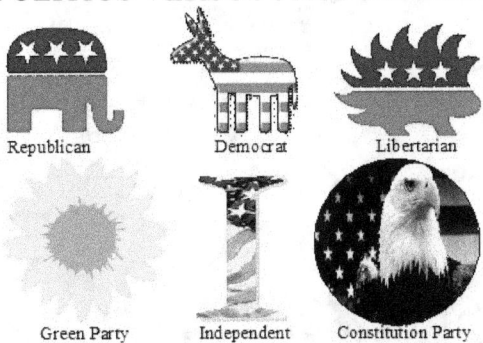

"Two subjects you must never discuss in general company; politics and religion." ~ Etiquette rule from 1879.

Though it will be a few years before you can vote (you're eligible at age 18), now is a good time to start thinking about how you will choose the officials who run your country. Most of the time, kids just go along with whatever political party their parents, neighbors and friends support. Politics tends to be a sensitive subject because many may have been raised to believe the opposing party is the "Evil Empire"; any politician on that platform must never be voted for, no matter what. Some may not even be aware that there are more than two parties to choose from! The danger with such ignorance is, so many people have no idea who they are voting for. Several years back, there was a story about someone who put a dog on the ballot – and the dog won! Far worse, what if an extremely corrupt person was running for office, and he was voted in not because of what he had accomplished, but because of his political party?

The wisest way to select officials is to find out who is on the bill, research the backgrounds of all the candidates, make your choices, then go to the polls to cast your vote. You can do this by typing "Sample Ballot" in a search engine, then enter your street address where it is indicated. As well as listing the people running for federal offices, it will list your state and local candidates. Feel free to engage your friends and family, and discuss your findings with them. Your sincerity in searching should prevent any arguments from erupting.

85

While reading, you may want to learn something about the type of work done while in office, so you will know if the entrants are realistic in their plans and, if elected, they are doing their jobs correctly. Who knows – you may decide you want to be in politics someday!

RELIGIONS VERSUS CULTS

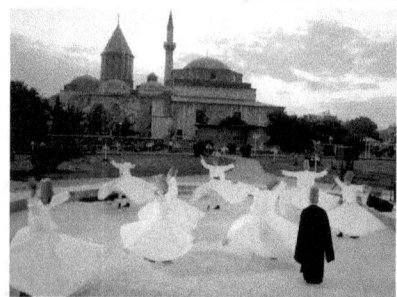

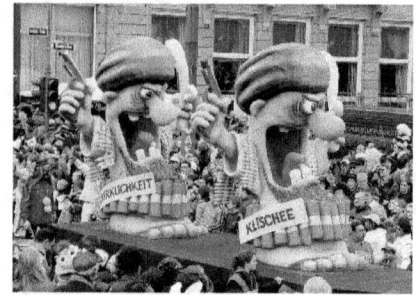

Whirling dervishes from the Sufi denomination of Islam. They take vows of poverty and humility, dedicating their lives to good deeds.

A float displaying Muslim suicide attackers. Though most Muslims are peaceful citizens, those few make Islam greatly feared today.

When choosing social groups, one must be careful – especially when it comes to religion! In the previous chapter, I mentioned a girl having a crush on a guy who lured her into dropping out of high school to join his Christian cult. In the past, cults were found mainly in countries with multiple ethnicities such as the United States, Australia, New Zealand and South Africa, but the internet has made it easy to recruit people from anywhere; as a result, they are now pervasive throughout the world. Often a cult will take out a page on social media, inviting people to join, and indoctrinating them that way. From there, local groups form where the new members meet. When it is discovered they are a cult, undergoing investigation by authorities as a result, they often deceive the public by changing their names.

While those based on religion are the most well known, other types exist that can be just as damaging:

Psychology: some primal therapy, designed to call up repressed memories, have been known to produce false ones, thus doing psychological damage and possibly ruining the reputations of innocent people.

Political: Many small extreme left or right wing political movements, which demand money, time, and absolute devotion of its members, are cults.

Corporate and Commercial: Several multi-level marketing companies are cults. They may hold seminars where members get hyped up emotionally to go out and make sales. In reality, very few people are successful in these ventures, since anyone can go to the nearest store and buy laundry detergent, vitamins, and makeup.

Scientific: These cults either use unethical means in their research and experiments, or steal the work of others and claim them as their own. The results, rather than presenting the truth, are skewed to suit their interests. An example is the recently popular low carbohydrate diet fad.

New Age: They promote expensive seminars that use deceitful means of recruitment, then brainwash people. EST from the early 1970s is a perfect example of this. It has since changed its name to The Forum, then Landmark Education; currently, it is called Landmark Worldwide.

Hate Groups: These proliferate in financially deprived sectors of society. During times and places of severe economic turmoil, such as pre-World War II Germany, they can take over entire countries. They function by blaming a certain group of people, based on ethnicity, social status, sex orientation, etc., for their troubles, believing that attacking them will improve their status.

Drug Cults: an example is Timothy Leary conducting his experiments with LSD in the 1960s. People involved in drug cults turn their bodies into laboratories, even chemical waste sites, without realizing what they're doing. The result is ruined health; it can also damage the brain to the point of being in a perpetually vegetative state. Total destruction or even death can happen the first time they try, depending on the drug, the substances mixed in, and the physical makeup of the user.

Cults based on religion, besides being the most well known, are also by far the greatest majority. An example of a religious cult is the Children of God (also known as The Family, or Family of Love). What makes joining such a cult particularly harmful is at the very least, it can waste valuable months or years of life, leaving former members disillusioned. With many, citizenship requires surrender of all money and worldly possessions to work for free (making the guru rich in the process – though the members don't know that). It is common for the cult master to have sex harems, including underage girls. If a severely restricted diet is one requirement (addling followers' brains so they can't reason correctly, which keeps them in the cult), it can threaten health. It can even put their lives in danger, if they're being enlisted or observed covertly by a criminal.

The most destructive cults are hate groups (examples are the Ku Klux Klan and inner city gangs). People who are lonely misfits or come from abusive backgrounds are most likely to be drawn to them. The cults come across as offering warm camaraderie, brotherhood and empowerment. They tend to be very sexist; they attract males through tactics such as video games with subliminal hate messages, relying on them to bring along their girlfriends (whose sole purpose is usually to breed for the cult). However, once the new initiate is trapped and vulnerable, they unleash a slew of abuse. They often require the convert to commit crimes to maintain membership; anyone who tries to leave is brutally murdered.

Currently, the cults that attract most media attention are extremist Islamic groups like ISIS and the Taliban. Fitting into both categories of religion and hate, they use techniques from the two camps; they approach disenfranchised people, discover what is important to them, and offer them just that. Often it is a humanitarian job, appealing to their idealism of making a world a better place. Women are lured with the possibility of dating and marrying a "good man". If the potential recruit is Muslim, they are told this is the true version of the religion, and currently they are at war with the corrupt variations of it. Once exposed to the cult's violent aspects, they are offered promises of elaborate rewards in the afterlife if they die for the cause; for instance, the Al Quaeda suicide attackers of the World Trade Center were told they would go to paradise and forever enjoy sensual pleasures with 72 vestal virgins. Martyrdom is hyped to the point where they can be classified as death cults; members are more interested in the afterlife than this one. Those who see through their guiles find it virtually impossible to escape, since they're most likely trapped in an isolated compound, often in a foreign country.

What makes cults especially insidious is that they are poorly understood. According to the dictionary, a cult is a religious group with practices that depart from what that particular faith considers the norm. How much they deviate is left up to interpretation, so this description is quite vague. It is commonly assumed that all cults consist of people who live restricted lifestyles in isolated communes under the rule of a harsh leader; in reality, most cult members live in their own homes, hold jobs, and visit church a few days a week. Another popular misbelief is that the only difference between a cult and a religion is about a million members. This came about because most religions got their start as tiny congregations that were suspected, even persecuted, by the majority. Judging a cult by its size is dangerously misleading, because some are very large with worldwide operations, while small but sincere worship groups are forced to deal with unmerited harassment.

To gain insight regarding cults, one must first understand religion, since the bulk of them spring from that base. The dictionary's definition of religion is a *cult*ure's system of social organization, practices, and world view. Religions are attempts to figure out how the world works, how to live the best life while here, and to explain the unexplainable such as what happens to us after we die. Thus, it provides civilization with a code of ethics. Superstitions develop when people don't understand the laws of Cause and Effect; an example is the Jewish / Islamic custom of avoiding "unclean" meats such as pork.

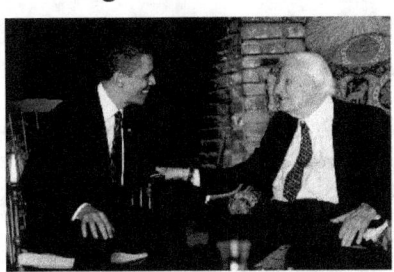

Billy Graham, world-respected Christian theologian whose ministry spans over 6 decades, meets with President Obama.

An estimated 4200 religions exist in the world today. The largest and most widely practiced ones are either Abrahamic or Hindu based. As scientific studies advance, many rationales behind religious practices are supported while others are proven obsolete. Example; pork can be safely consumed if cooked thoroughly to kill the cause of trichonosis, thus doing away with the belief that it is "unclean". Some religions readily accept scientific discoveries that go contrary to their teachings, while other cling tightly to tradition, fearing nasty repercussions from a mysterious cosmic source for deviating from age-old conventions. Many faiths forbid its members to learn about other modes of worship; some even frown on associating with another denomination!

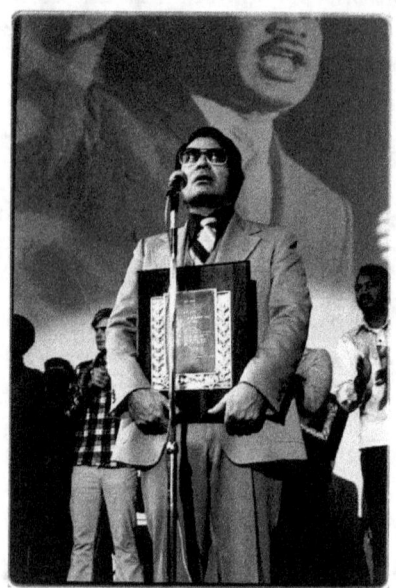

Jim Jones, founder of the cult Peoples Temple, accepts the Martin Luther King award less than 2 years before his death in the largest mass suicide in American history.

This is why religion lends itself so well to cults. While all world religions have cult offshoots, Christianity and Islam, due to their belief that they have Absolute Truth, produce the most. *A cult is basically a mind control vehicle.* It lures followers by preying on their insecurities, presents them with an instantly formed family and community, and charms them with the belief that they are a special elite group as opposed to the "sinful world". They provide a pseudo-shelter in an environment that seems terrifying. They feed their congregation false promises of prosperity in the next life for obeying its outlandish rules, threatening them with horrific consequences if they don't comply.

Who joins cults? What's really scary is that enlistees are not feeble-minded or lacking in intelligence. They are perfectly normal; what makes them different is that they had the misfortune of coming across a particularly seductive recruiter at a critical time in their lives. People are most vulnerable to joining cults when they are experiencing a major transition, such as moving out on their own, which is why most cult neophytes are in their late teens / early 20s. However, everyone experiences a major life change at one time or another, whether it be relocating hundreds of miles away, altered health or financial status, getting married / divorced, even aging.

Also, coming from a dysfunctional family can drive a young person to seek acceptance and love by joining a cult. Some, like the late River Phoenix, were raised in one, having no choice in the matter.

So how can you avoid being hoodwinked?

First, be aware of religion's true role. As I stated earlier, ethnicities all over the Earth built their belief systems on their understanding of how the world works. In other words, all creeds are a form of ancient science. Their purpose is to enhance the lives of followers. Any restrictions it places on them are supposed to be for their own good. It is one thing to frown on adultery; it is quite another to force people to suppress sexuality altogether. Forbidding wasted time in idleness is understandable, but when they demand devotees work constantly, never taking time out for harmless pleasures, this is when the religion becomes over-controlling. If it fills up with lots of superfluous rules with no solid reasoning supporting them, this is a sign the religion itself could be a cult.

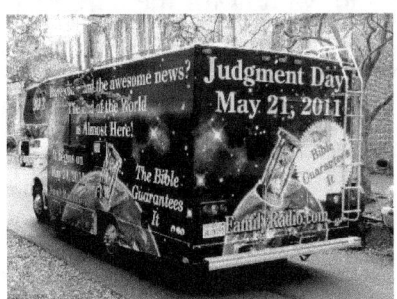

Would you give up your life savings to join a doomsday cult? How about your iPod music library? Or submitting to censor-ship of innocent pastimes like dancing, movies or reading fantasy novels?

Second, recognize what a cult looks like. Cults tend to have 3 traits. They are 1) exclusive; "We're the only ones with the Truth; everyone else is misinformed" (how likely is that with the world population topping 7 billion?): 2) secretive. Few people in the cult know what's really going on; only the ones in the upper echelons of the society know (greatly enabling corruption!): and 3) authoritarian. You obey the leader without question. The worshipped Deity could be a currently living person, or someone from the distant past for whom the guru serves as a "spiritual messenger". Commonly cults have strict rules regulating behavior, dictating what emotions to feel, labeling some (usually erotic desire, skepticism and anger) as "evil", and requiring followers to contort themselves to doing something unrealistic such as instantly forgiving someone who molested them as a child. Many control what types of literature members may read and music /

shows to enjoy. Some go so far as to place tremendous pressure to marry in haste and have large families the couples can't afford (though they use flattery towards this end, the real goal is to enlarge the cult through breeding). Almost universally, they use hypocritical means to mislead: for example, they will come up with arguments that have pre-set answers, giving the illusion of allowing questioning; they tell you they accept all religions, while either bashing the others or declaring themselves superior; they point the finger at other creeds that either have worse reputations or more oppressive regimes ("We're not a cult; they are!"); or they may break their own rules by severely restricting sexual activity, yet allow for "flirty fishing" (attracting new converts by having sex with them). Anyone who sees some things that are amiss is admonished to not point them out. If they do, they will either be told to ignore it, given some vague answer or scolded for being "apostate".

Third, remember you live in *this* world! Religion is supposed to enhance your life, not confine you while waiting for the hereafter. Ultimately, beliefs regarding what happens when our time on Earth is through are mere speculations; the only ones who really know are those who have had near-death experiences, and even then, that is their individual adventure. Some cults, preying on people's fear of living, encourage members to escape the world; they may require them to dress in outdated fashions, even banning technology, with the strong message that the "Good Old Days" were less sinful. They're assured there's no need for them to be aware of current events; it's none of their concern. They can just float in this sanctified cocoon until Judgment Day. This may seem comforting, but it renders them ill-prepared for life; if they leave, either through their own volition or because the cult fell apart, it could have severe repercussions, to the point of becoming homeless. A religion with true wisdom will be a positive guide for the only existence you can know, which is the here and now. Any charlatan can promise pie-in-the-sky; in this case, if their assurances prove to be false, you may not be able to reclaim what you lost.

Having a loved one in a cult is the acme of frustration. Because many cults discourage members from associating with outside family and friends, lest doing so causes them to "backslide", the new recruit usually abandons them. Unfortunately, not much can be done about this, because the person is brainwashed. Definitely do not bluntly confront them! They have already been programmed to see this as "persecution"; they will give you a coded answer and cut you off. The only thing you can do is try your best to stay close, restricting your conversation to non-controversial subjects. If they try to convert you, calmly listen and ask questions that will guide them to see the faults in the cult's logic. They must find out the truth for themselves; no one can tell it to them. The good news is, most cult recruits eventually discover it's a farce and leave on their own; typically after a year. That is the time they will most need support from their loved ones; definitely be there for them then. Do not judge; remember, anyone can be enticed into a cult! The only difference between you and a cult member is circumstance!

This leads to the complication of how to escape a cult. Fortunately, for most people, it's just a matter of making up one's mind. It may not be easy because of losing the social structure the cult provided, plus lingering fears the guru could be right, but it is possible. The problem lies with those that belong to a cult that allows only one way out, which is a protracted painful death. Those cases usually require law officials knowledgeable about the situation to work with the person. Gang members who want to leave could get themselves arrested, transported to a jail far away, then released. In the case of an Islamic cult, more drastic measures have to be taken. In some cases, people have faked their own deaths.

Members isolated in a commune are very difficult to rescue; they may have to be kidnapped, which means if they don't have outside friends and family members aware of their situation, they could be doomed. It is for this reason that, above everything else, you must *NEVER* go to a "retreat" sponsored by a group you know nothing about! It is significant that Jim Jones of the People's Temple cult waited until everyone was trapped in Guyana, South America, before launching his horrific abuse. Out of the near thousand people in Jonestown, only 87 escaped the mass suicide.

Whole books have been written on the nature of cults, but this should at least give you an idea of how they work. While it's true that anyone can be vulnerable, your best defense is to be open-minded and tolerant. The easiest people to recruit into a religious cult are those who have determined there is only one way to think. If you're convinced a church exists that has Absolute Truth, all a cult recruiter has to do is tell you he belongs to that church and extend an invitation; you attend a few meetings and are love-bombed into accepting their doctrine. If you're already in "such a church", a recruiter can agree with you, then say you need to tweak your program a bit; you can do that by joining his group; this is the way David Koresh of the Branch Dividians gathered members. It is also important to learn about other world religions, which will give you wisdom to recognize an imposter. With over 7 billion people on Earth spread out over 6000 languages and ethnic groups, there is no need for bigotry; any Deity worth worshipping will welcome the various styles of devotion from all of mankind. If you harbor any doubts regarding this, survey the state of the world and ask yourself what sort of parent you would be if you ran your home in such a chaotic, narrow-minded way.

Ultimately, developing discernment to choose friends and associates wisely, whether live or in cyberspace, religious or secular, is a tremendously important skill. There is a saying, "The company you keep will affect and influence the opportunities you meet"; this is very true. The people you surround yourself with can make or break you. Good social skills are among the most important traits you can have!

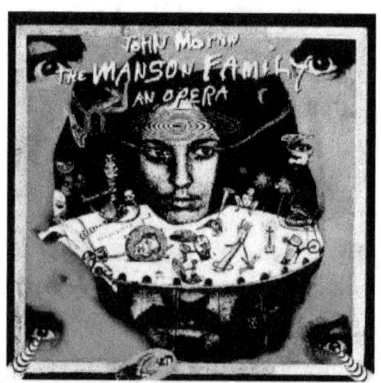

"A long habit of not thinking a thing wrong
gives it a superficial appearance of being right."
~ Thomas Paine

Conversion

1) A cult member once told me about a fellow believer who went out with a man she met on an internet dating site. He slipped her a date rape drug, and she awoke abandoned in her car several hours later. The man disappeared; since his profile was fake, the law was unable to trace him. (This is one major reason why high school kids should not use internet dating services – it's risky enough for adults, even!) She blamed it on the woman taking personal responsibility to find a partner, rather than trusting God to do so.

   She said the woman went on to give birth to a "lovely girl" with severe autism, prone to extreme violence to the point where she could not be around other children. (Can you see her faulty logic here?)

   Hold a group discussion on ways she could have protected herself from becoming a crime victim, *AND* what she should have done in the event it didn't work (for starters, when she awoke in her car, she should have immediately gone to the hospital without cleaning up or anything else, and demanded a rape kit with emergency contraception). This is important to know, because anyone can be slipped a date rape drug; it doesn't have to come from someone you met on the internet.

2) To help you decide which political party to vote for to serve as President, take this online quiz. https://www.isidewith.com/political-quiz

   Afterwards, read thoroughly about the recommended Presidential candidate. If everyone based their votes on such research, think of how much better off America would be!

3) Read the history of a famous cult, such as Branch Dividians or a more extreme one like Al Quaeda, and study their recruiting techniques. Obviously people don't deliberately choose to isolate themselves in an abusive

95

environment or become suicide bombers. How did these cults lure them into doing so?

4) Read about other world religions so you can gain insight regarding their perspectives. Here are some links to get you started.

What Takes More Courage Than Rebellion?
Considering Another Point of View

Part I: Abrahamic Religions
http://hubpages.com/religion-philosophy/What-Takes-More-Courage-Than-Rebellion-Considering-Another-Point-of-View

Part II: Hindu-Based Religions
http://hubpages.com/religion-philosophy/Considering-Another-Point-of-View-Part-II-Hindu-Based-Religions

Part III: Far East Asian Religions
http://hubpages.com/religion-philosophy/Considering-Another-Point-of-View-Part-III-Far-East-Asian-Religions

Part IV: Combined Religions
http://hubpages.com/religion-philosophy/Considering-Another-Point-of-View-Part-IV-Combined-Religions

While reading about your religion, try to view it objectively, as someone from another faith would see it.

What do all of them have in common?

Can one solve a particular problem, such as a chronically poor social sector, better than the others?

Note that each one started in a different place and time. What does that say about any religion having Absolute Truth?

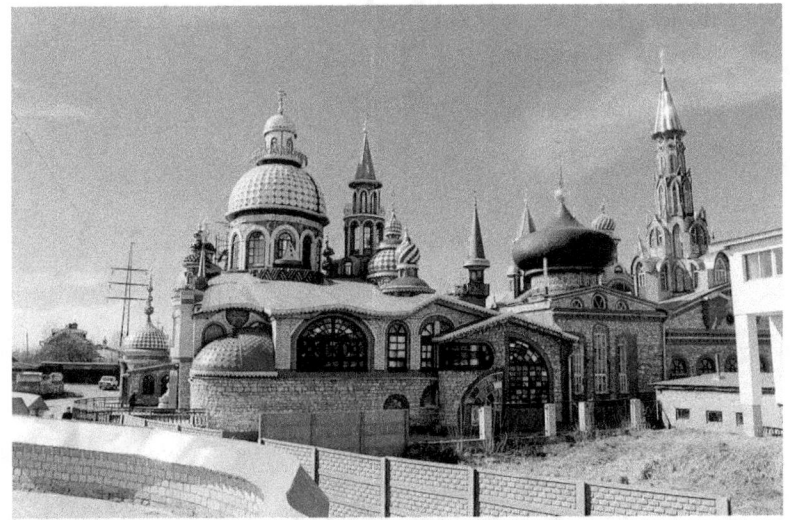

Temple of All Religions in Kazan, Russia

Religious Pluralism – your best defense against cults!

CHAPTER FIVE

RESPONSIBITLY AND PREVENTION PART III

SEXUALLY TRANSMITTED DISEASES

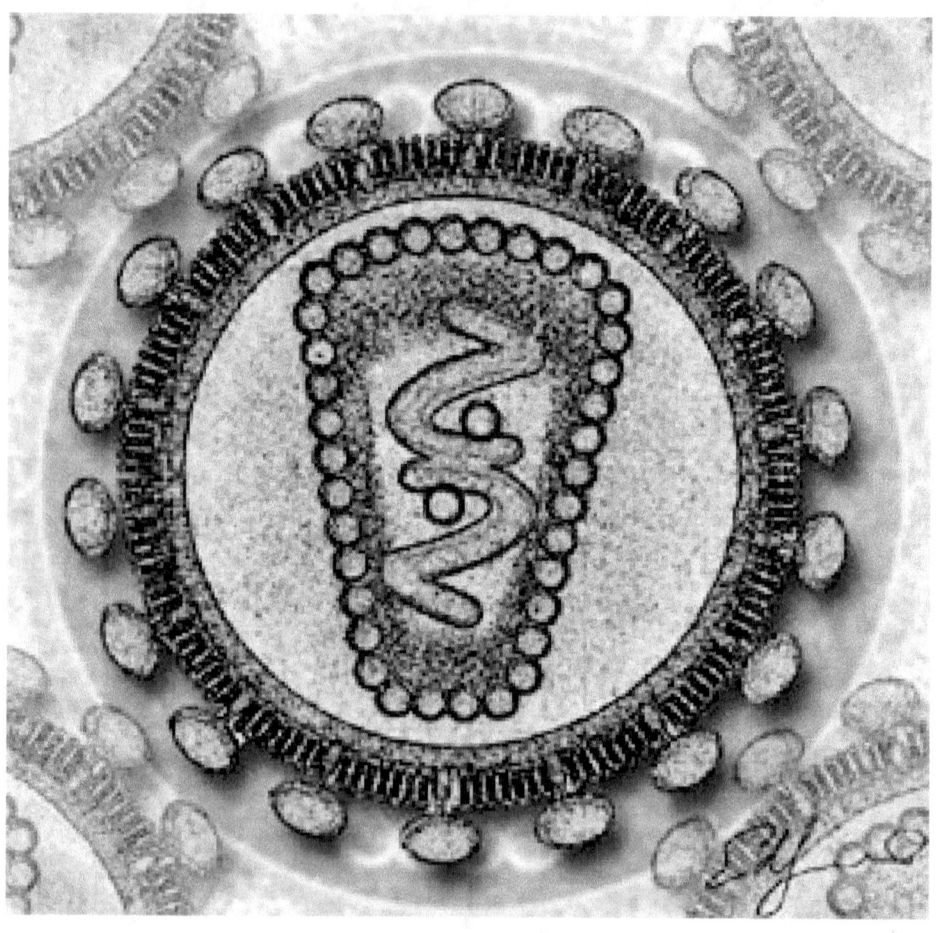

Human Immunodeficency Virus - Stylized Rendering

Ask Pointed Questions:

Identify which of these statements are myths, and which ones are true.

1) Proper condom use prevents transmission of all sexually transmitted diseases.

2) A person with no obvious herpes sores can't transmit the virus to his or her partner.

3) Only homosexuals have to worry about HIV, the virus that causes AIDS.

4) Guys don't have to worry if they get HPV (genital warts), since it causes cancer only in girls.

5) Sexually transmitted diseases nearly always have symptoms, so you know if you've contracted one.

6) Bacterial infections, such as chlamydia and gonorrhea, can easily be treated with home remedies, and may even go away on their own.

7) Having sex in a hot tub will kill bacteria and viruses that cause sexually transmitted diseases.

8) You cannot get a sexually transmitted disease from oral sex.

9) You can't have two or more sexually transmitted diseases at the same time, and you cannot be re-infected with a particular sexually transmitted disease once you contract it.

10) One night stands are safe, since sexually transmitted diseases are relatively rare.

Answers: All are myths.

Though having a good sex life produces many benefits, it does have a negative side. Over 20 diseases are spread this way, some of which are incurable, and may even result in death. The couple could also be saddled with babies they may be ill-prepared to care for. It is these reasons sex has acquired a negative reputation, since it is only within the past century that cures and prevention became known. Before these discoveries, abstinence was the only real way to avoid problems.

In this and the next chapter, I will address both concerns. It's a good thing we live in an age when the vast majority of issues can be dealt with, and even avoided!

Sexually transmitted diseases are also referred to as STDs, STIs (infection), and the old fashioned term venereal diseases (named after Venus, the Roman Goddess of Love). They are mainly spread through penis / vagina, oral, and anal intercourse; some can also be contracted other ways. I will list here the most common diseases in order of occurrence, along with photos of what the bacteria / virus looks like (I am also adding links to several, in case you want to look at gross pictures of symptoms). I have included the chances of getting infected in the form of how many sex partners one has, but bear in mind you can only catch an illness from someone who has it; this means you could have thousands of partners and never get one, or you may become afflicted with an extremely rare condition from your very first encounter.

Disease: **Cytomegalovirus (CMV)**

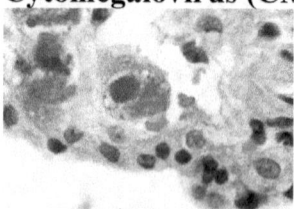

Symptoms: CMV is related to herpes. In most people, there are no symptoms. On rare occasions, one may suffer fever, sore throat, enlarged lymph nodes, appetite loss, fatigue, and achy muscles. In someone whose immune system is suppressed,

100

the virus can attack various organs throughout the body, causing diarrhea, pneumonia, hepatitis, vision loss, even seizures and coma. Most babies born with CMV exhibit no symptoms; however, 20% may experience jaundice, low birth weight, skin rash, pneumonia, enlarged liver / spleen, and seizures.

Other Ways Contracted: Virtually anyone can contract CMV. It is spread through contact with blood, semen, vaginal secretions, breast milk, saliva, and urine. This means kissing, blood transfusions, organ transplants, and sharing needles can spread it, as well as breastfeeding. Most babies born to infected mothers don't have the virus; out of those who do, only 1 – 2% will develop problems as a result.

Chances of Contracting: 1 – 2 partners.

Treatment / Cure Rate: There is no cure. People who suffer from resulting diseases, or are at risk, such as recent transplant patients, are placed on an antiviral regimen. Fortunately, most people with CMV need no treatment.

Disease: **Herpes**

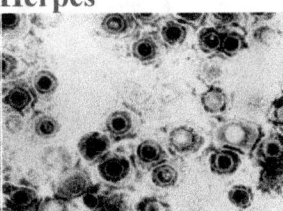

https://commons.wikimedia.org/wiki/File:Herpes_labialis.jpg

https://commons.wikimedia.org/wiki/Category:Herpes_genitalis#/media/File:SOA-Herpes-genitalis-female.jpg

https://commons.wikimedia.org/wiki/Category:He
rpes_genitalis#/media/File:SOA-Herpes-genitalis-
male.jpg

Symptoms: Painful blisters near the mouth or in genital area. The person can spread it by touching the sores and then the eyes or other areas with mucous membrane without washing hands.

Other Ways Contracted: Herpes is spread through sex and French kissing. Less commonly, it can be contracted through sharing eating utensils and drinking glasses. (Other forms of herpes, such as Chicken Pox and Shingles, are contracted through ways other than sex.)

Chances of Contracting: 5 partners.

Treatment / Cure Rate: There is no cure, but medications can reduce symptoms and likelihood of passing it on. If a woman has an outbreak while giving birth, she will need to have a C-section to avoid infecting her baby.

Disease: **Intestinal Parasites**

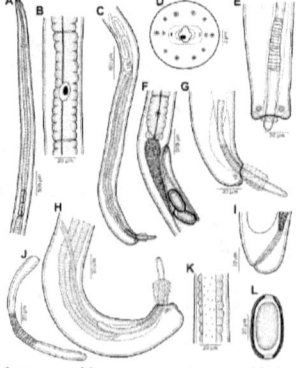

https://commons.wikimedia.org/wiki/File:Parasit
e140131-fig2_Capillaria_plectropomi
(Nematoda)-_Scannin_Electron_Microscopy.tif

Symptoms: In most cases, the disease is Giardiasis, Amebiasis, or Cryptosporidiosis. The incubation

102

period is 2 – 3 weeks, and often there are no symptoms; the parasites can exist in the body for years. Symptoms, when they occur, are diarrhea or constipation, cramping, allergies, gas / bloating, anemia, chronic fatigue, ulcers, and irritable bowel syndrome.

Other Ways Contracted: These types of parasite infections are transmitted via the fecal / oral route; through ingesting contaminated water or food handled in an unsanitary manner. Sexually, it can be contracted through analingus or rimming (tongue to anus), fellatio after anal sex, and putting anything in the mouth – sex toys, fingers, etc. – after insertion in the anus.

Chances of Contracting: 6 partners.

Treatment / Cure Rate: Giardiasis and Amebiasis are 100% curable; doctors treat with antibiotics. Cryptosporidiosis is not curable; however, medications used to treat Giardiasis show promise. Untreated, intestinal parasites can lead to chronic food allergies, lactose intolerance, and immune system dysfunction. Amebiases can cause dysentery, which may lead to death.

Disease: **Mycoplasma Genitalium**

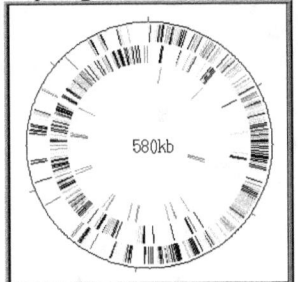

Symptoms: In men; watery discharge from penis. In women; abnormal vaginal discharge, and bleeding in between periods, especially after sex.

In both; pain and discomfort when urinating.

**Other Ways
Contracted:**   It is spread only through sex.

**Chances of
Contracting:**   14 partners

**Treatment /
Cure Rate:**   It is 100% curable with antibiotics. Untreated, it can lead to urethritis, miscarriage, pre-term birth, Pelvic Inflammatory Disease, and infertility.

Disease: **Chlamydia**

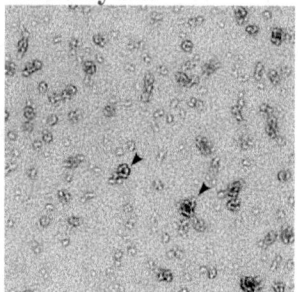

https://commons.wikimedia.org/wiki/Category:Chlamydia_infections#/media/File:SOA-Chlamydia-trachomatis-female.jpg

https://commons.wikimedia.org/wiki/Category:Chlamydia_infections#/media/File:SOA-Chlamydia-trachomatis-male.jpg

Symptoms: Unusual discharge from the vagina, penis, or rectum; burning pain when urinating; rectal pain and bleeding; painful swelling of testicles. Often there are no symptoms, but the disease still causes damage, so sexually active people should get tested regularly.

**Other Ways
Contracted:**   It is spread only through sex.

Chances of Contracting:	37 partners.
Treatment / Cure Rate:	It is easily cured through antibiotics. Be careful to take them as the doctor orders, and wait 1 week after the last dose to resume sex. Untreated, it can lead to infertility and ectopic pregnancy in women, and a constricted / blocked urethra in men.
Disease:	**HPV (human papillomavirus, aka genital warts)**

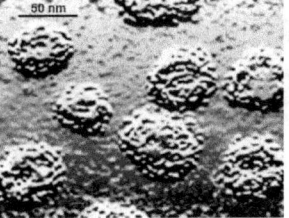

https://commons.wikimedia.org/wiki/Category:Genital_warts#/media/File:SOA-Condylomata-acuminata-female.jpg

https://commons.wikimedia.org/wiki/Category:Genital_warts#/media/File:SOA-Condylomata-acuminata-man.jpg

Symptoms:	Over 120 types exist; 15 are known to be carcinogenic. Symptoms are cauliflower like warts in the throat and genital area. Most of the time, there are no symptoms, and most people who have it are unaware. It can be passed with by people with no symptoms.
Other Ways Contracted:	It is spread only through sex.
Chances of Contracting:	50 partners.

Treatment / Cure Rate:	Most cases go away with no treatment; the ones that don't may go on to cancers of the cervix, vulva, penis, anus, and throat. Vaccines exist for the most virulent strains; 6, 11, 16, and 18. They are administered in 3 doses over the course of 6 months, and should be received before people become sexually active.

Disease: **Crabs (Pubic Lice)**

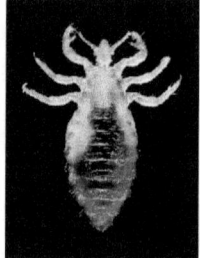   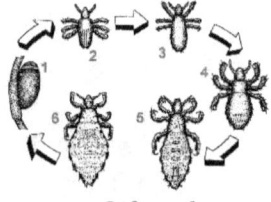

Adult louse   *Life cycle*

https://commons.wikimedia.org/wiki/File:SOA-Pediculosis-pubis.jpg#/media/File:SOA-Pediculosis-pubis.jpg

Symptoms:	Tiny insects and eggs in pubic hair, black spots on underwear, and hives / itching in the affected area. Scratching can cause inflammation and sores, which may become infected.
Other Ways Contracted:	Most cases are through sexual contact; however, using towels, sleeping in sheets, and wearing clothing that contains lice and their eggs can cause it. The lice may spread to any area that has hair, such as eyebrows, eyelashes, the scalp, even all over the body. However, it is *NOT* transmitted through pets; lice specifically need a human host to survive.
Chances of Contracting:	90 partners.

Treatment /
Cure Rate: It is 100% curable. The affected area should be washed with a lice-killing shampoo that contains 1% Permetherin. If more than one treatment is needed, wait a week before trying again. All nits (lice eggs) must be removed by combing or being pulled out by hand, since they are not killed by shampoo. Applying olive oil makes it easier to comb the nits out.

As well as killing the lice, all clothing and bedding used by the patient must be washed in hot water. What cannot be washed must be dry cleaned and placed in tightly-sealed plastic bags for two weeks, to suffocate the lice and nits (lice eggs).

All sex partners within the past month need to be notified and contacted. Sexually activity should resume only after cure is complete.

Disease: **Hepatitis**

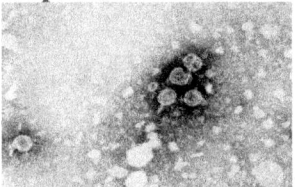

https://commons.wikimedia.org/wiki/Hepatitis#/
media/File:Jaundice_eye.jpg

Symptoms: This is a liver disease. Though there are several strains (from A to G), A, B, and C are the most common forms that are sexually transmitted. Symptoms are fatigue, fever, appetite loss, achy muscles and joints, pain in abdomen, nausea / vomiting, and jaundice (yellowing of skin and eyes). Often there are no symptoms; most people who have it are unaware of their condition.

Other Ways Since Hepatitis is a virus spread mainly through blood, it can also be contracted by sharing needles,

107

Contracted: toothbrushes and razors, blood transfusions, non-hygienic body piercings / tattoos, and unsanitary health care practices. Hepatitis A can come from food and water contaminated by raw sewage, and contact with feces of an infected person. Hepatitis B can come from other bodily fluids besides blood, such as semen and vaginal fluids.

Chances of Contracting: 100 partners.

Treatment / Cure Rate: A and B can be prevented through vaccines; Hepatitis C can't. Treatments for Hepatitis C continue to advance; starting treatment early has led to an 80% cure rate, but the costs run tens of thousands of dollars. Ultimately, Hepatitis C can lead to liver cancer and death. Hepatitis A usually heals on its own; Hepatitis B may do so, but can also become chronic, in which case it could lead to liver cancer and / or cirrhosis of the liver.

Disease: **Trichomoniasis**

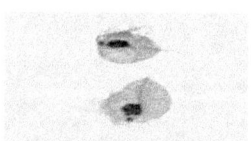   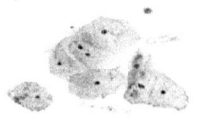

Trichomonas Protozoa   *Pap Smear Test Result*
https://commons.wikimedia.org/wiki/File:Tricho monas_vaginitis_5241_lores.jpg

Symptoms: This infects the woman's vagina and the man's urethra. Only 30% of people experience symptoms. They include burning painful urinating, irritation and inflammation of the sex organs, penile secretion, and unusual smelling discharge from the vagina.

Other Ways Contracted: It is spread only through sex.

Chances of Contracting: 100 partners

Treatment / Cure Rate: It is 100% curable. Not getting treated makes sex painful, and the sufferers more vulnerable to other STDs. Women are more prone to miscarry or experience preterm birth.

Disease: **Lymphogranuloma Venereum (LGV)**

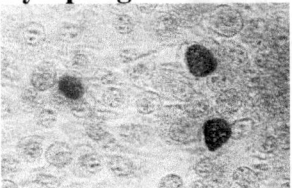

https://commons.wikimedia.org/wiki/File:Lymp hogranuloma_venerum_-_lymph_nodes.jpg#/media/File:Lymphogranulo ma_venerum_-_lymph_nodes.jpg

Symptoms: LGV is a form of chlamydia, in which the bacterium enters through a break in the skin. The first symptom is easy to miss; it is a painless sore at the site of entry, which usually heals within a few days (it is even more difficult for women to locate, since it often occurs in the interior of the vagina). The secondary stage causes painful swelling in the lymph nodes.

Other Ways Contracted: It is contracted exclusively through sex.

Chances of Contracting: 110 partners.

Treatment / Cure Rate: If caught early, it is 100% curable, though recurrences often happen. It is treated with a 3 week course of antibiotics; sometimes, the swollen glands have to be lanced. All sex partners from the previous two months must be contacted, and sex should not be resumed until course is complete. Untreated LGV may lead to

109

elephantiasis of the genitals, fistulas in the sex organs, and strictures / scarring of the rectum which can cause death. If LGV goes systemic, it can cause arthritis, hepatitis, perihepatitis, and pneumonia.

Disease: **Gonorrhea**

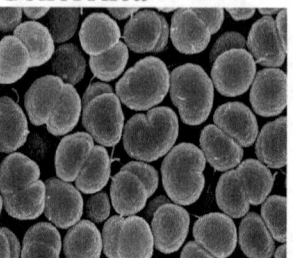

https://commons.wikimedia.org/wiki/Gonorrhoea#/media/File:SOA-gonorroe-female.jpg

https://commons.wikimedia.org/wiki/Gonorrhoea#/media/File:SOA-gonorroe-male.jpg

Symptoms: Painful burning urination; yellow, green or white discharge from the penis or vagina; bleeding between periods; swollen painful testicles; anal discharge, itching, soreness and bleeding; pain when moving bowels. Often, gonorrhea has no symptoms at all.

Other Ways Contracted: It is spread only through sex.

Chances of Contracting: 141 partners.

Treatment / Cure Rate: Completely curable, but it is very important to take all your medication as the doctor prescribes, since drug-resistant strains exist. Untreated, it can lead to pelvic inflammatory disease, ectopic pregnancy, and infertility in women, and blocked urethra and infertility in men. In both genders, it can spread to the joints and the bloodstream, in which case it can cause death.

Disease: **HIV /AIDS (human immunodeficiency virus / acquired immune deficiency syndrome)**

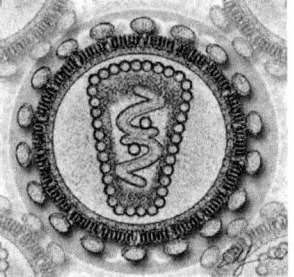

https://commons.wikimedia.org/wiki/File:Kaposi%E2%80%99s_sarcoma_intraoral_AIDS_072_lores.jpg

Symptoms: Often there is no initial evidence of infection. About a month after exposure, some people experience flulike symptoms. They go away and the patient enters the latency stage, in which he or she remains symptom free as long as 10 years, but the destruction of the immune system continues, during which the person can spread the virus. The disease then progresses to AIDS, in which the patient experiences strange cancers, pneumonia, tuberculosis, and a variety of neurological disorders.

Other Ways Contracted: It is spread through sex, but any exchange of the bodily fluids blood, semen, breast milk and vaginal secretions can pass on the virus. This includes sharing needles and rinse water from injected drug use, and – rarely – from blood transfusions, tissue transplants, and pre-chewed food from an infected person. A pregnant woman may pass the virus to her unborn baby; taking antiretroviral meds, having a C-section and avoiding breastfeeding reduces this risk.

Chances of Contracting: 300 partners.

Treatment / While there is currently no vaccine or cure, great advances have been made regarding treatments.

Cure Rate: People in high risk groups for exposure can take a medication called PrEP (Pre-Exposure Prophylaxis), which prevents the virus from taking hold in the body. Those who have already been exposed can take PEP (Post-Exposure Prophylaxis) up to 72 hours after exposure, greatly reducing the chance of HIV developing into AIDS. People who already have AIDS can maintain their immune systems by taking medications as the doctor prescribes, and practicing healthy living habits.

Disease: **Molluscum Contagiosum**

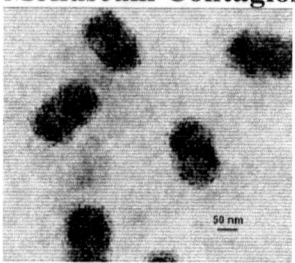

https://commons.wikimedia.org/wiki/Category: Molluscum_contagiosum#/media/File:Molluscal klein.jpg

Symptoms: The disease is caused by the poxvirus. Symptoms are lesions, white or flesh-colored, with a dimple in the center. They are painless, but may itch. They form anywhere on the body, but rarely on the palms of hands or soles of feet.

Other Ways Contracted: Molluscum contagiosum is easily transmitted by skin-to-skin contact, and sharing towels / bedding / clothing. The lesions can spread by touching them, then other parts of the body. For this reason, it is best to avoid scratching the lesions, and to keep them covered with band-aids.

It can possibly be transmitted in a swimming pool, though this is rare. It is most common among children under age 12; older patients usually get it through sexual contact.

Chances of Contracting: 100 – 1000 partners. Since many people don't seek treatment, exact figures are uncertain.

Treatment / Cure Rate: Molluscum contagiosum is relatively benign. In most cases, it clears on its own within 6 to 12 months; however, it could take up to 4 years. In most cases, no scarring occurs, but scratching could cause scarring. In severe cases, the doctor treats it with a cream / liquid or by freezing the lesions, scraping them off, or burning them through chemical treatments.

Though molluscum contagiosum is caused by a virus, it does not stay in the body, so the patient can contract it again.

Disease: **Scabies**

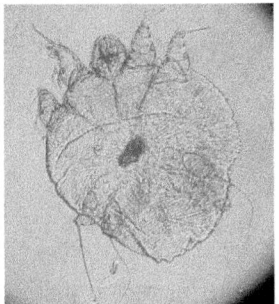

https://commons.wikimedia.org/wiki/File:Acaro dermatitis_Hand.jpg#/media/File:Acarodermatiti s_Hand.jpg

Symptoms: The disease is caused by a mite that burrows into the skin and lays its eggs there. Symptoms are red rash and severe itching, which tends to get worse at night. It can occur anywhere on the body. Scratching can break the skin, allowing infection to enter. In severe cases crusting occurs, though this is often due to poor hygiene and a weak immune system.

113

Other Ways Contracted: In adults, it is almost exclusively through sex. However, prolonged skin-to-skin contact, and sharing towels / clothing / linens with an infected person spreads it. It is most prevalent in crowded depressed areas such as slums and refugee camps. The mite is human-specific, so it cannot be transmitted through pets.

Chances of Contracting: 1000 partners.

Treatment / Cure Rate: It is 100% curable, with the use of medicated creams. All bedding and cloth items used within the past 3 days should be washed in hot water and dried in a dryer. All sexual contacts within the past month should be notified and receive treatment.

Disease: **Mononucleosis ('Mono')**

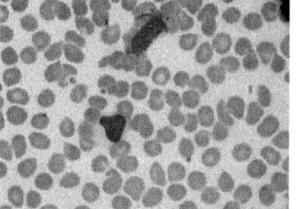

https://commons.wikimedia.org/wiki/File:Mono nucleosis1.jpg

Symptoms: Fatigue, malaise, inflamed tonsils, sore throat, strep that isn't healed with antibiotics, achy muscles, swollen spleen, fever, headache, rash. Symptoms usually come a month to 6 weeks after exposure.

Other Ways Contracted: Through kissing, sharing eating and drinking utensils, even being near a patient who coughs or sneezes - though it's not as contagious as the common cold.

Chances of Contracting: 2000 partners.

Treatment / Cure Rate: Mononucleosis (nicknamed the "kissing disease") is caused by the Epstein-Barre virus. Usually it clears up on its own; if symptoms continue longer than a week, it is time to see a doctor. Severe cases can lead to ruptured spleen, hepatitis, swollen heart valves, breathing troubles from tonsils blocking airway, encephalitis and meningitis. Doctors treat it with corticosteroids and antibiotics; the regimen depends on the symptoms and degree of severity the particular patient suffers. Currently, researchers are working on a vaccine. Since it is caused by a virus, most people do not get the disease twice; however, on rare occasions, an immunocompromised person can come down with it again.

Disease: **Syphilis**

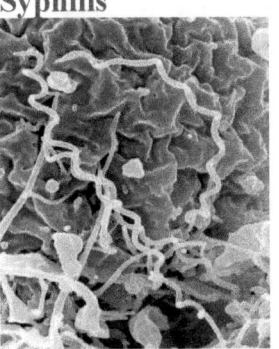

https://commons.wikimedia.org/wiki/Category:Syphilis#/media/File:Extragenital_syphilitic_chancre_of_the_left_index_finger_PHIL_4147_lores.jpg

https://commons.wikimedia.org/wiki/Category:Syphilis#/media/File:2ndsyphil1.jpg

https://commons.wikimedia.org/wiki/Category:Syphilis#/media/File:A_case_of_tertiary_Syphilis_to_the_back_Wellcome_L0038263.jpg

Symptoms: Symptoms come in 3 stages. Primary: a painless chancre sore at site of introduction, which goes away after about a month. Secondary: lesions in mouth and sex organs, skin rashes, patchy hair loss, flulike symptoms, fatigue, and weight loss. Latent / Late: this may occur up to 30 years after infection. It includes neurological disorders, mental illness, blindness, and death. Pregnant women may miscarry or experience stillbirth, or pass the disease to their infants, producing birth defects.

Other Ways Contracted: It is spread almost exclusively through sex. However, it can be transmitted if broken skin comes in contact with a chancre sore. Mothers can also pass it on to their babies during pregnancy or childbirth.

Chances of Contracting: 10,000 partners

Treatment / Cure Rate: Syphilis is 100% curable; however, it is important to get treatment as early as possible, since whatever damage has occurred cannot be reversed.

Disease: **Chancroid**

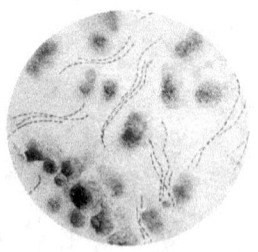

https://commons.wikimedia.org/wiki/File:Chancroid_lesion_haemophilus_ducreyi_PHIL_3728_lores.jpg#/media/File:Chancroid_lesion_haemophilus_ducreyi_PHIL_3728_lores.jpg

Symptoms: Painful, pus-filed ulcers in the genital area. This is often accompanied by swollen lymph nodes. The sores can become infected, and make it easier for the patient to contract HIV.

Other Ways Contracted: It is contracted almost exclusively through sex, though health workers may be infected by working with patients, since it is spread through skin contact.

Chances of Contracting In western countries; 1.9 million partners. In developing countries, infection is far more likely; in fact in some areas, Chancroid is more prevalent than herpes. Sex trade workers are particularly vulnerable.

Treatment / Cure Rate: It is easily cured with antibiotics. The patient takes it for 1 – 2 weeks. Neglecting treatment can cause Phimosis, which is scarring and thickening of the foreskin requiring circumcision, and superinfection that may make it necessary to debride the inguinal lymph nodes.

The following diseases are contracted, in addition to sex, by neglecting treatment of existing STDs and poor health practices.

Disease: **Bacterial Vaginosis**

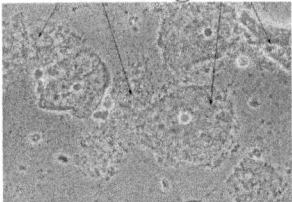

Symptoms: Only women get this disease. The balance of normal bacteria in the vagina is upset, causing symptoms of itching and burning in the vaginal area, and a fishy smelling discharge which may be gray or white in color. Many women have no symptoms.

Other Ways Contracted: Caused by sex and douching.

117

Chances of Contracting: Having even one partner can cause it. If the woman douches, she can get it without a sex partner.

Treatment / Cure Rate: Completely curable. Sometimes it heals itself, though treatment is advisable. Having BV may lead to premature birth, make women more vulnerable to other STDs, and even cause PID.

Disease: **Yeast Infection**

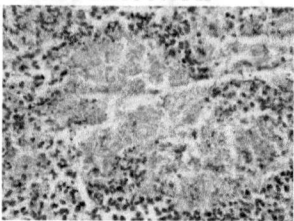

Symptoms: Technically, this is not considered an STD, though it can be contracted through moving any object from anus to vagina, having sex with an infected partner, and receiving oral sex from someone with thrush. Symptoms are vaginal discharge that is a whitish-gray color; it is usually thick, though in some instances it can be watery. The penis produces a whitish discharge in the skin folds, and the head may become inflamed. Other symptoms are rash, burning, itching, soreness, and painful sex.

Other Ways Contracted: Wearing tight clothing made of synthetic fabrics that don't ventilate well, douching, using feminine deodorant sprays, prolonged sitting in a hot tub of water, wiping from back to front after defecating, and infrequent changing of feminine products. Uncircumcised men who practice poor hygiene are more prone to yeast infections, and people who suffer from diabetes, are overweight, use antibiotics for a prolonged period or have a suppressed immune system are also vulnerable.

Chances of Contracting:	The number of partners has no direct effect, though the more a person has, the greater likelihood they'll get a yeast infection.
Treatment / Cure Rate:	It is 100% curable through medications. Usually a doctor prescribes it in cream or pill form; patients who gets it often can find ways to treat it themselves. If a woman has a chronically recurring case – 4 times a year or more – her diet may be causing a bacterial imbalance in her vagina, in which case she needs to eat a lot of yogurt or take a supplement containing lactobacillus. Men can treat it with over the counter antifungal medications.
Disease:	**Urethritis / Urinary Tract Infection**

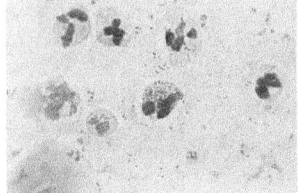

https://commons.wikimedia.org/wiki/File:Neutro phils_phagocytizing_bacteria.jpg

https://commons.wikimedia.org/wiki/File:SOA-non_specific_Urethritis-female1.jpg

Symptoms:	Urethritis is infection / constricting of the urethra, the tube through which urine passes out of the body. Urinary tract infection is an invasion of bacteria inside the bladder itself. There are three types of Urethritis; **Gonococcal** which is caused by gonorrhea, **Nongonococcal (NGU)** which caused by an STD other than gonorrhea (Chlamydia, in most cases), and the one caused by something other than an STD, such as trauma from catheter insertion. All types, plus UTI, have the symptoms of burning

119

pain while urinating, discharge from urethra, itching, tenderness, irritation, and stains on underwear. Urethritis has a greater incidence in men because they are more likely to have symptoms of gonorrhea and chlamydia. Women, on the other hand, are more prone to urinary tract infections because their urethras are shorter (2 inches, as opposed to 8 inches in men).

Other Ways Contracted: Urethritis can also be caused by trauma from inserting a catheter, urinary tract infection, irritation from spermicide or other chemical, phimosa (tightening of the foreskin), urethral stricture, reactive arthritis and inflamed prostate gland. Urinary tract infections in women can be caused by wiping back to front after defecating.

Chances of Contracting: Since both are often caused by untreated STDs, the number of partners has no direct effect, though the more partners one has, the greater the likelihood of contracting either one. Low-functioning immune system, and menopause in women, can make one more vulnerable to UTIs.

Treatment / Cure Rate: They are 100% curable with antibiotics. What is prescribed depends on the cause. If untreated, symptoms may go away after 3 months, but person remains infected and can spread it. Untreated urethritis can lead to pelvic inflammatory disease, blocked urethra, and sterility in both genders. Untreated UTIs can lead to sepsis and kidney failure.

Disease: **Pelvic Inflammatory Disease**

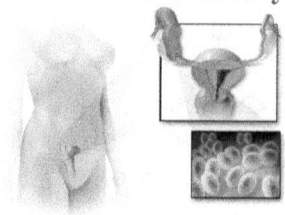

120

Symptoms: Though mainly suffered by women, men can get this too. Symptoms are fever, lower abdominal pain, foul-smelling vaginal discharge, burning painful urination, painful sex, and between-period bleeding.

Other Ways Contracted: PID is caused by untreated chlamydia or gonorrhea. It can also be contracted through douching and using an IUD.

Chances of Contracting: The number of partners has no direct effect, though the more a person has, the greater likelihood they'll get an STD that can lead to PID.

Treatment / Cure Rate: It is 100% curable through medications. The earlier it is caught, the better the chances of avoiding permanent damage. Untreated, it may cause chronic pelvic pain, urethral stricture in men making it difficult or impossible to urinate, and scar fallopian tubes leading to ectopic pregnancy or sterility in women.

The incidence of these diseases can be reduced with condoms. It is important to use them correctly, to minimize their failure rate. Also realize that some diseases, such as herpes and HPV, have viruses so small they can pass through condom pores. Ultimately the best prevention is knowing your partner well and staying monogamous.

121

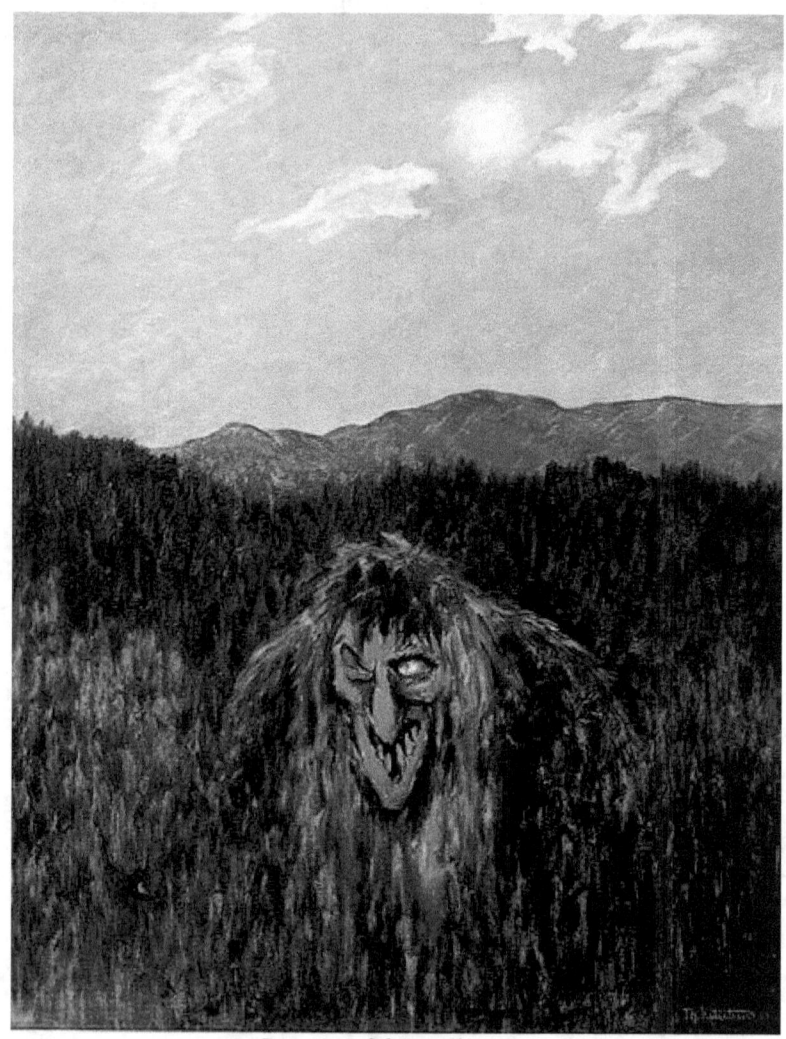

Beware of the troll!

The Real Deal:

1. A common belief is that religion and various authority figures suppress sexuality. Make a list of ways they do this, then write the reasons why they may or may not have a point with these restrictions.

2. A person diagnosed with an STD is told to inform all partners, so they can be tested and treated. Though this can be awkward and embarrassing, it is necessary. Syphilis was a common STD 40 years ago; today, it has been nearly eradicated. Discuss ways someone can explain to a partner they have an STD, especially if it's an incurable one like herpes or HBV. Hint; they can tell their partner what they're doing to control outbreaks, and how they plan to avoid passing it on.

CHAPTER SIX

RESPONSIBILITY AND PREVENTION PART IV

BIRTH CONTROL

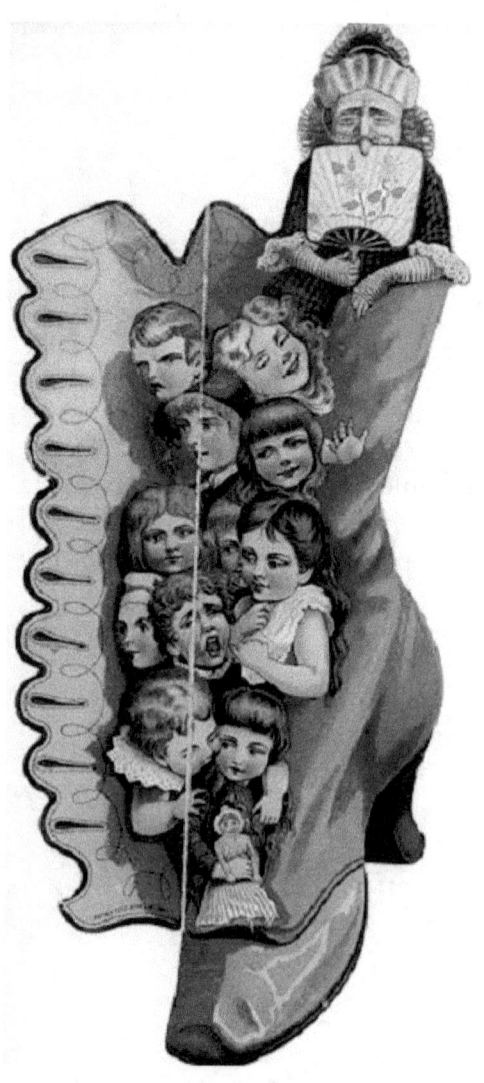

"There was an old lady who lived in a shoe.
She had so many children, she didn't know what to do."

Go Over with a Fine-Tooth Comb:

Identify which statements are myths, and which ones are true.

1) Birth control methods have been used since antiquity. The reason poor families were larger than wealthy ones in the past is because wealthy people were more educated in such matters.

2) Having sex in the standing position is one way to prevent pregnancy.

3) A girl can't get pregnant the first time she has sex.

4) A girl can't get pregnant if she has sex while on her period.

5) Using birth control, rather than dampening sexual enjoyment, actually enhances it.

6) If a couple is short on condoms, they can rinse it out and re-use it.

7) If a couple doesn't have a condom, a baggie or plastic wrap can be an equally effective birth control method.

8) Douching with Coca Cola is a valid form of birth control, since it will kill sperm.

9) When choosing a method of birth control, the person's health must be taken into consideration, since some methods can exacerbate problems while other methods can relieve or prevent them.

10) Condoms are the only form of birth control that protects against sexually transmitted diseases.

Answers: 1, 5, 9, and 10 are correct;
2, 3, 4, 6, 7 and 8 are myths.

125

n the past, concerns about unwanted pregnancy hampered enjoyment of sex. A few methods of birth control were available through the forms of ingesting special herbs, wearing crude condoms, and practices such as avoiding sex during particular times in the woman's cycle. However, most of the knowledge was lost to the Western world during the Medieval Age when Bubonic Plague was rampant and the birth rate needed to be high as possible to keep the population from dying out. When Margaret Sanger opened America's first birth control clinic in 1916, it was still considered a controversial subject; many people believed God should decide the size of families, not humans.

The facts are, most people engage in sexual activity for reasons other than procreation, and families are healthier when children are born by choice rather than by chance. Thank goodness birth control options have greatly improved through quality as well as quantity! Here is a list of them, in order of effectiveness.

Method: **Abstinence**

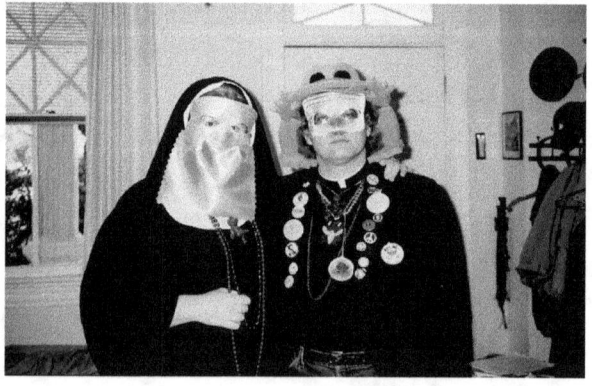

This is refraining from penis / vagina intercourse. "Outercourse", such as mutual masturbation, can be done in its place. Some people also engage in oral or anal sex.

Advantages: It is the only form of contraception that is 100% effective. If sexual activity is avoided altogether, it allows for the couple to truly get to know each other, since sex doesn't get in the way. Immature people should avoid sex until they're ready to handle the responsibilities.

Disadvantages: This is unrealistic for couples in serious, long term relationships. Historically, it has promoted discrimination against women, purporting they must be virgin brides and keep out of public while men visited prostitutes for release. Also, while this prevents pregnancy, STIs can still be spread through oral and anal sex.

Method: **Sterilization**

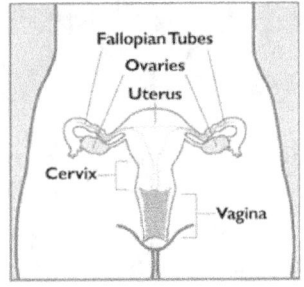 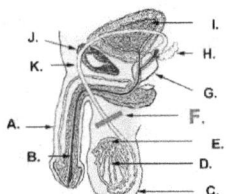

Surgically cutting or blocking the fallopian tubes of the woman (called tubal ligation) prevents the egg from entering the uterus. When it is done to the vas deferens in the man (vasectomy), his ejaculate doesn't contain sperm. It is almost 100% effective.

Advantages: One procedure lasts for life; the couple never has to worry about birth control again. It does not change hormone balance, and has no side effects.

Disadvantages: Another form of birth control must be used for 3 months while the sperm is cleared from the ejaculate or new tissue grows around the blockage. Though the surgery is safe, there is always a possibility of complications, such as the fallopian tubes growing back together and causing an ectopic pregnancy. Most important of all, the surgery is irreversible. There are exceptions, but it is best undertaken by people who are sure they want no children in the future.

Method: **Implant**

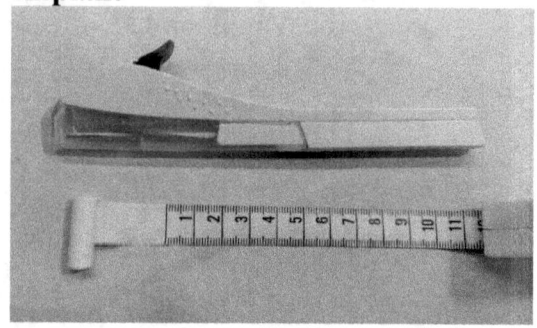

A flexible plastic piece the size of a match is placed underneath the skin of the woman's upper arm by a doctor. It releases hormones that prevent ovulation and thickens cervical mucus. It lasts 3 years and is over 99% effective.

Advantages: Because it lasts so long, the couple doesn't need to worry about doing anything else for birth control. The woman can become pregnant immediately upon removing the Implant, and it can be used by those who cannot handle estrogen or are breastfeeding.

Disadvantages: The Implant cannot be used by breast cancer patients. Other than that, side effects are rare and minimal. The most common are changes in menstrual cycle. Most women have lighter, fewer periods; some stop having them altogether. In a few cases, they can become heavier, with spotting in between. If infection or jaundice occurs, consult a doctor immediately.

Method: **Intra Uterine Device**

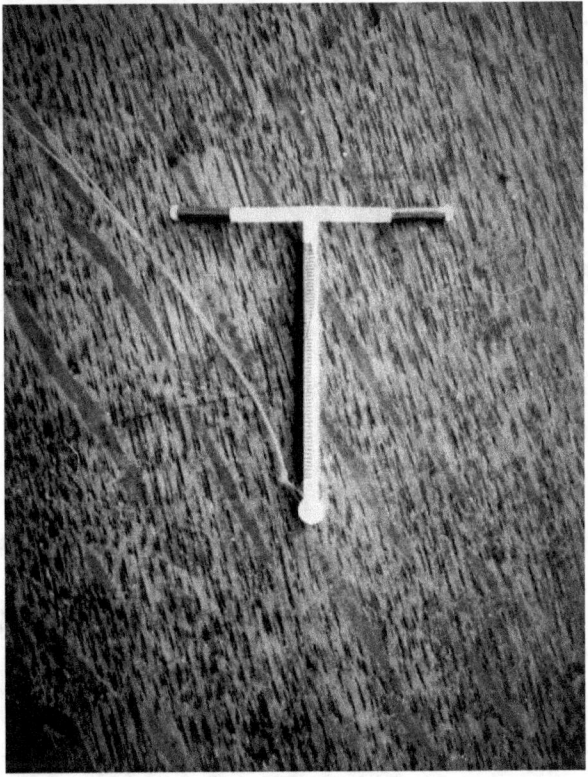

The doctor implants a device in the woman's uterus, which prevents the egg from being fertilized. A hormonal IUD can block the egg from being released. It is over 99% effective.

Advantages: IUDs have become much safer over the years. As a result, they are less likely to cause heavy bleeding and cramps; some brands actually reduce them. Women can breastfeed while using an IUD, since it doesn't interfere with her hormonal balance. She can get pregnant immediately after it is removed. There are no worries about usage, and it allows her to be spontaneous.

129

Disadvantages: While IUDs are much safer than they used to be, they still carry many risks. They may perforate the uterus, or slip out; both need immediate medical attention. They can cause an ectopic pregnancy, and pelvic inflammatory disease. Though IUDs are generally effective immediately, some may not work until one week after insertion, depending on when they were placed during the woman's cycle. Women who have cancer of the breast, cervix, or uterus, liver disease, a recent history of PID or pelvic tuberculosis, or may be pregnant should not use an IUD. Those who have Wilson's Disease or are allergic to copper should not use ParaGard.

Method: **Breast Feeding**

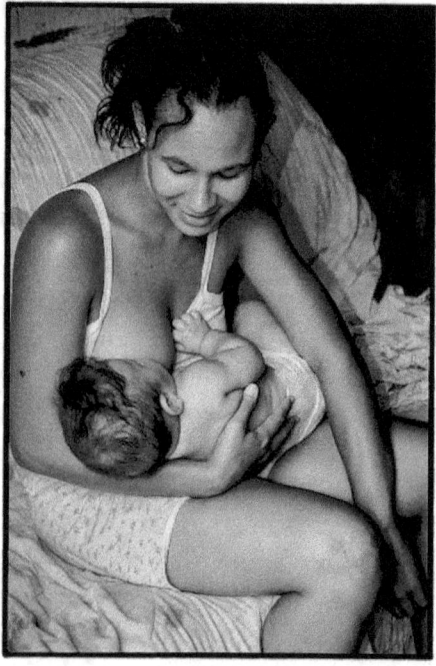

This is an ancient method of birth control. If a new mother breastfeeds her baby every 4 hours during the day and every 6 hours at night, her body refrains from producing hormones that promote pregnancy. Effectiveness is about 98%.

Advantages: This method has many advantages. There are no side effects, it is free and requires no prescription, and it has multiple health benefits to both the mother and the baby.

Disadvantages: It works for only 6 months, the program must be followed exactly in order to work, and it can be inconvenient to maintain the schedule. It may lessen vaginal moisture, and some women feel less sexual when breastfeeding.

Method: **Injection**

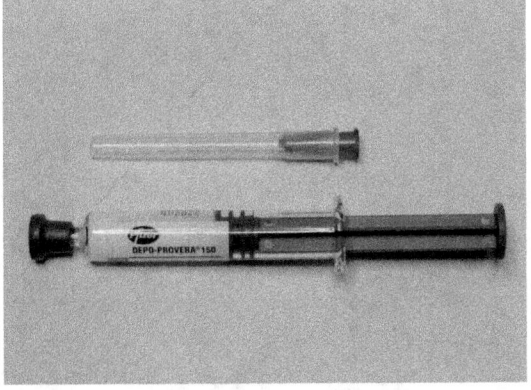

The woman gets a shot of progestin hormone. This blocks ovulation and thickens her cervical mucus, so sperm cannot reach the uterus. It is 99% - 94% effective, and works for 12 weeks.

Advantages: It is convenient; no pill or procedures to remember, since it is done only every 12 weeks, so it promotes spontaneity. A woman can also maintain her privacy, since she doesn't have to carry anything. Since it contains no estrogen, it can be used by those who have issues with the hormone, and may help prevent uterine cancer.

131

Disadvantages: The Injection has multiple side effects; depression, weight gain, longer heavier periods with spotting in between, hair loss or Hirsutism, tender breasts, nausea, headache, and sex drive change. Unfortunately, little can be done about the side effects; they must be endured until the medication wears off. Women who experience migraines, jaundice, pus, bleeding at injection site, pain that lasts several days, and develop a new breast lump should consult their doctors immediately. Those who have breast cancer, Cushing's disease, osteoporosis, or may be pregnant should not get the Injection.

Method: **Vaginal Ring**

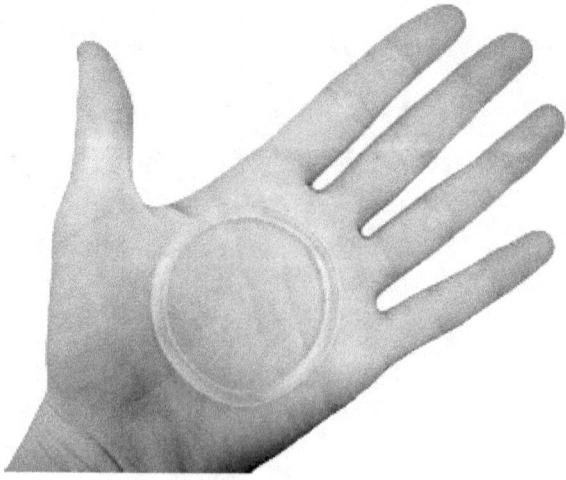

A flexible ring is placed into the vagina once a week for 3 weeks, then left out for 7 days. It releases hormones that prevent ovulation and thickens cervical mucus. It is 99% to 91% effective.

Advantages: Since it is inserted once a week for 3 weeks, there is little to worry about. In addition to birth control, it helps cure acne, bad cramps, osteoporosis, cancers of the ovary and endometrium, PID, PMS, and anemia. It can also prevent ectopic pregnancy and non-cancerous breast cysts and tumors.

Disadvantages: Women who are prone to migraines, heart disease, cancer, blood clotting disorders, have diabetes, liver disease, must spend a lot of time in bed, have weak pelvic floor muscles or are pregnant should not use this method of birth control.

Method: **Birth Control Pill**

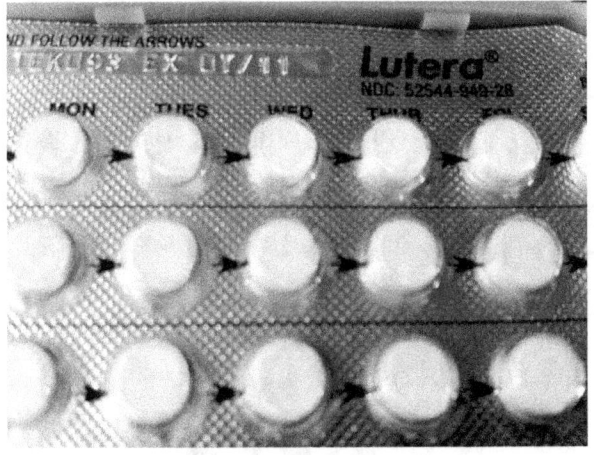

There are two main types of this hormone treatment; estrogen and progesterone (regular); and progesterone only (mini pill). The doctor decides what to prescribe, according to the woman's needs and physiological makeup. It works by blocking ovulation, and preventing sperm from entering the uterus by making the cervical mucus thicker. Its effectiveness ranges from 99% - 91%.

Advantages: The Pill is taken once a day, then no more worries. It regulates erratic periods, reduces

133

cramps, and lightens menstrual flow. It can protect against osteoporosis, ectopic pregnancy, acne, anemia, benign breast tumors, cancers of the ovary and endometrium, pelvic inflammatory disease, and breast and ovarian cysts.

Disadvantages: The Pill must be taken at the same time every day, in order to work. If a pill is missed, another form of birth control must be used for a week. Some antibiotics and medications that treat seizures, fungal infections, and HIV, and herbs like St. John's Wort, may render it ineffective. Side effects may include nausea / vomiting, spotting between periods, tender breasts, depression, and change in sexual desire. The woman must wait for at least 2 months after ceasing usage to attempt pregnancy. Birth control pills are discouraged for women who have breast cancer, heart disease, diabetes, lupus, liver disease, uncontrolled high blood pressure, or smoke.

Method: **The Patch**

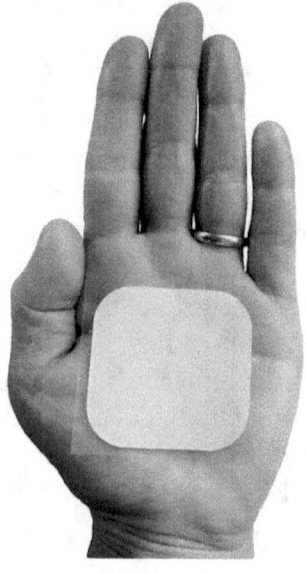

134

A thin patch which releases the hormones progestin and estrogen is placed on the woman's skin. It is replaced every 7 days for 3 weeks, then left off for a week. It blocks ovulation, and thickens cervical mucus to prevent sperm from entering the uterus. It is 99% to 91% effective.

Advantages: The woman only has to think about it once a week. It also has the advantages of regulating periods and relieving severe cramps, PMS, reproductive tract cancers and infections, anemia, acne, benign tumors and cysts, and osteoporosis.

Disadvantages: The Patch may cause skin irritation. If the woman forgets to change it on schedule, or if it falls off, she needs to use another form of birth control for a week. Certain medications that treat HIV, fungal infections, seizures, and antibiotics may render it ineffective, as does St. John's Wort. Women who get migraines, are pregnant, smoke and have high blood pressure or are over 35 years of age, have liver disease, diabetes or lupus, or with a history of heart disease, liver or breast cancer, blood clots or stroke should not use the Patch.

Method: **Diaphragm**

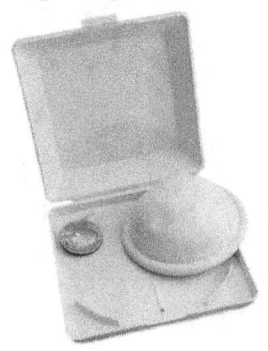

This is dome with a flexible rim that fits over the cervix, blocking sperm from entering the uterus. It must be used with a spermicide, and the woman needs to be fitted for one by a doctor. Its effectiveness ranges from 94% to 88%.

Advantages: It is easy to carry, and is relatively inexpensive to get. It can be reused, and once in place, can be utilized for multiple sex acts.

Disadvantages: It can be difficult to insert, and can be pushed out of place by heavy thrusting and some sex positions. If the woman has a significant weight change, she may need to be refitted for one.

Method: **Sponge**

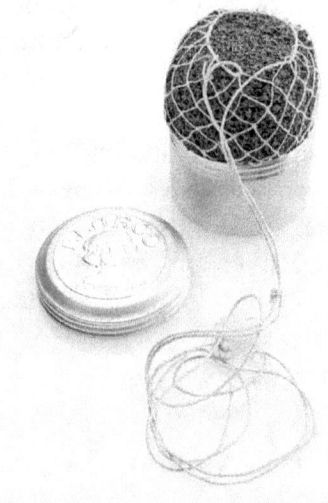

A 2 inch piece of plastic foam treated with a spermicide is soaked with water and inserted into the vagina up to 24 hours before intercourse. It must be left in for 6 hours after the last time the woman has sex. Effectiveness is 92% - 88%.

136

Advantages: Easy to use and carry around, does not interfere with sex, cannot be felt by either partner, can be used for multiple sexual acts, can be used while breastfeeding since it does not alter the woman's hormones.

Disadvantages: Can be difficult to insert or remove, can cause vaginal irritation and dryness, partner could have sensitivity to spermicide. If sponge breaks apart in the vagina, a doctor may need to remove all the pieces.

Method: **Emergency Contraception**

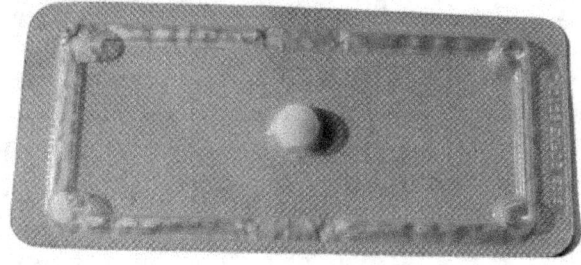

This can be used up to 5 days after intercourse. It comes in 2 types: pills, 1 or 2 are taken, and intrauterine device, inserted by a doctor. It is 85% effective. The IUD remains effective for up to 12 years.

Advantages: It is safe to use, and a good backup system in the case of unexpected intercourse.

Disadvantages: Because of its low rate of effectiveness, this is best used only in emergency cases rather than as a regular form of birth control. It is less effective in overweight women, even those with a BMI as low as 25. Side effects include nausea / vomiting, dizziness, breast tenderness, and irregular periods.

137

Method: **Condoms**

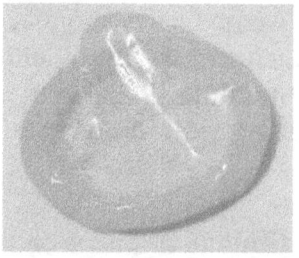

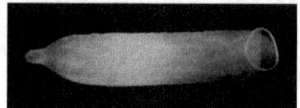

*Female
Condom*

Male Condom

This is a sheath that covers the penis, preventing sperm from entering the uterus. Condoms have been used since antiquity, made out of materials varying from specially treated linen cloth to animal intestines; they were reusable. Today, they are made of plastic or latex, and are to be used only once per sex act. There is a female variety as well as the traditional male; unlike the male, the female condom can be inserted at any time. Male condom effectiveness ranges from 98% to 82%; female ranks slightly lower, from 95% to 81%.

Advantages: Condoms are the only form of birth control that protects against sexually transmitted diseases. They are inexpensive and easy to get and carry around. Putting them on can be a form of foreplay, and some men are able to maintain erection longer and avoid premature ejaculation while using them. The female condom remains in place even if the man loses his erection, and the outer ring can stimulate the clitoris. Condoms can be used for oral and anal sex as well. Many come in varying textures and flavors; some even glow in the dark!

138

Disadvantages: Condoms can be irritating for people who are allergic to latex; they should use plastic ones instead. Some people complain it cuts down on sensations. Some find it cumbersome to put on a male condom after erection and before intercourse.

Method: ## Natural Family Planning

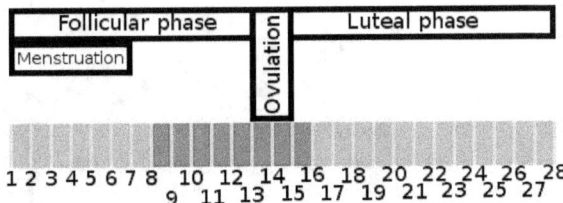

Risk of conception:
∎ : risk
▨ : no risk

Follicular phase | Ovulation | Luteal phase
Menstruation

1 2 3 4 5 6 7 8 10 12 14 16 18 20 22 24 26 28
9 11 13 15 17 19 21 23 25 27

The woman's cycle is charted so the couple knows when she is fertile, and avoids sex during that time. This method is ancient; in the past, it was done by keeping track of her periods to time her ovulation, and checking her cervical secretions (the mucous becomes clear and slippery mid-cycle). Today, in addition, her temperature is measured daily (it spikes during her most fertile time), Its success rate ranges from 98% to 76%.

Advantages: It is safe to use; since no medications are involved, there are no side effects or conflicts. The costs are low; the couple only needs to buy calendars, thermometers, and charts. They can quit anytime, and can strive for pregnancy soon as they stop.

Disadvantages: NFP does not work for women who have irregular periods. It is cumbersome to keep track of so many factors, since even if periods are regular, cycles vary slightly from month to month. This is especially true for a woman who is going off birth control pills, is a teenager, is breastfeeding, or approaching menopause. A major problem of following the program exactly is that a woman often gets her strongest sexual urges during her fertile time. Her partner needs to be fully committed to the program, and classes need to be taken to learn proper procedure.

Method: **Withdrawal**

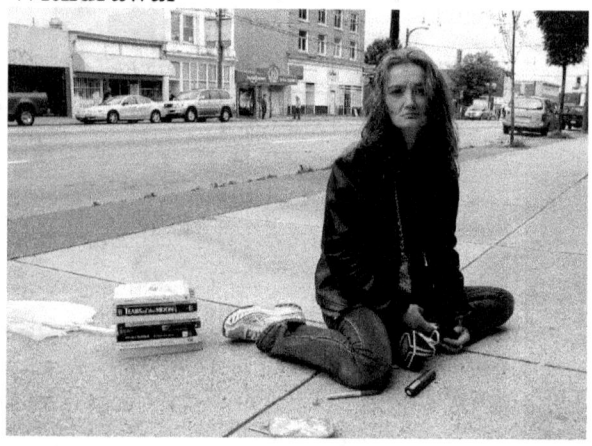

(No, I don't mean withdrawal from drugs, but that must be what it feels like). This is one of the world's oldest forms of birth control. Just before ejaculating, the man withdraws his penis from the woman's vagina. Effectiveness ranks from 96% down to 73%.

Advantages: It is free, doesn't require a doctor visit, and has no medical side effects.

Disadvantages: It requires a tremendous amount of self-control, and is not for men who are sexually inexperienced or suffer from premature

140

ejaculation. It has a high failure rate. It doesn't protect against STIs.

Method: **Spermicide**

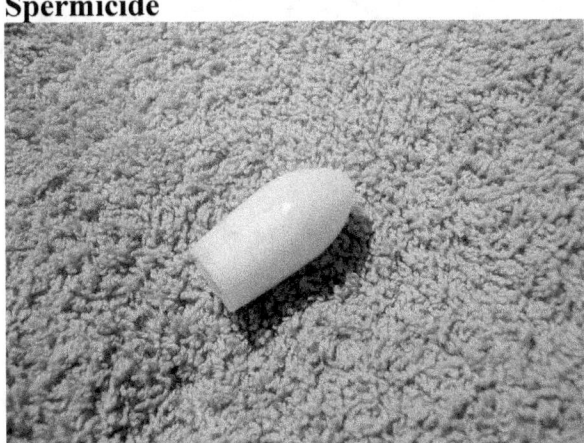

Though many barrier methods contain spermicide, it can be used by itself. However, effectiveness is significantly less; 82% - 72%. The foam or gel is inserted into the vagina, and the woman must remain in a reclining position so it doesn't slide out. Spermicide kills and immobilizes sperm.

Advantages: It can be easily carried around, can be bought in most stores, since it does not alter a woman's hormones she can use it while breastfeeding, and it can be part of foreplay.

Disadvantages: It has a high failure rate, and can cause irritation to the penis and vagina. It must be inserted 10 minutes before intercourse, must be renewed before each act, and remains effective for only an hour afterwards.

Method: **Cervical Cap**

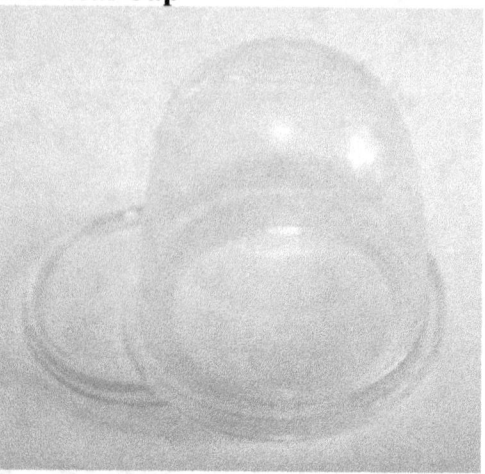

This is a silicone cup placed over the cervix, to block sperm from entering the uterus. The woman needs a doctor's visit to be fitted for one. It must be used with a spermicide, and its effectiveness ranges from 86% to 71%.

Advantages: It is convenient to carry, and to use. Once in place, it can be left in for up to 6 hours, and is good for multiple sex acts. Since there are no hormonal effects, it can be used while breastfeeding.

Disadvantages: Using the cervical cap is not advised for women who have given birth within the past 10 weeks, or have had a recent abortion, cervical surgery, are on their periods, have allergies to spermicide or silicone, have cancer of the vagina, vulva, or uterus, an infection in the reproductive organs, toxic shock syndrome, or any other problem such as poor vaginal muscle tone. It may be pushed out of place during sex, and it is more expensive than the diaphragm.

The next two methods I will list separately, because of their great possibility to be detrimental.

Douching. The purpose is to wash the sperm out of the vagina, before it enters the uterus. Not only does it work poorly (possibly facilitating pregnancy by forcing sperm into the uterus), it can be downright harmful. Douching can bring on ectopic pregnancy and pelvic inflammatory disease. If Lysol is used, it can even kill the woman through poisoning.

Abortion. This is best used only under the direst circumstances. Perhaps the couple was immature or ignorant, the prophylactic method failed, the baby was conceived under negative circumstances or has a disability, or the pregnancy is dangerous to the mother. If an abortion is performed within the first trimester, it is actually safer than bearing the child to term; however, there is no advantage of using it as a form of birth control. Not only does it carry risks similar to any other operation, but multiple abortions may weaken the cervix, rendering the woman unable to bear children to term in the future, and damages the psyches of all involved.

These topics are very important because the more knowledge people have, the better they are able to make responsible choices. Ultimately, the best-lived life is achieved by those most informed – and prepared.

Your Take On It:

1. Perhaps you find birth control too cumbersome to use. In that case, you should figure out what type of parent you would make, since 85% of couples who have unprotected sex become pregnant within a year. Here are a couple of online quizzes, for starters.

    http://www.gotoquiz.com/will_you_be_a_good_parent

    GoToQuiz complies with the Digital Millennium Copyright Act (DMCA).

    Created by: donttellmyname

    http://www.allthetests.com/quiz31/quiz/1409243432/Would-you-make-a-good-parent

    10 Questions - Developed by: Dauna Quimby - The quiz is developed on: 2014-09-01

    While you're at it, bear in mind that in the US, it costs an average of $245,340 dollars to raise a child to age 18. That doesn't account for factors such as living in an expensive place like New York or the San Francisco Bay Area, or if the pregnancy is difficult, the birth has complications, or if the child is handicapped. You may decide birth control isn't so cumbersome, after all.

2. In the mid-1990s, when very little could be done about AIDS, a woman with the disease was told by her doctor she had 2 years to live. She was living on public assistance, and had 3 children (by 3 different men), all of whom she was neglecting. In spite of this, she decided she wanted to have another baby. The man who impregnated her contracted HIV during the process, thus obtaining a death sentence from her; as you can see, this issue affects men as well as women, even though men don't get pregnant.

    Today, some countries and certain parts of the United States consider exposing someone to HIV a felony, tantamount to homicide. It is punishable by hefty fines and a prison

144

sentence.   Other areas consider it a misdemeanor; but wherever it happens, the offender can be sued.   Even back when this story took place, the man could have hauled the woman to court.   Obviously though, it would have done him no good; even if she had any assets, all the money in the world wouldn't have restored him to health.   This explains why it is vital to know your partner well before having sex.

She quite possibly also passed the virus on to her baby.

Discuss the ethics of bringing a life into the world when the parents have nothing to offer it.   How would you feel if you were that baby?

CHAPTER SEVEN

MAKE ROMANCE + FINANCE = TRANSCEN-DANCE

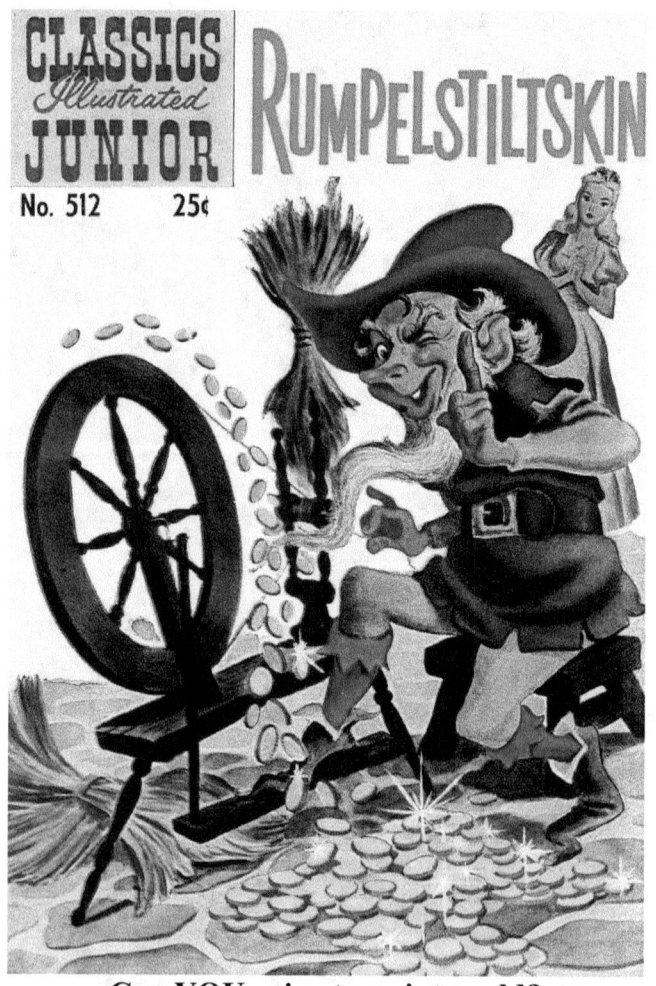

Can YOU spin straw into gold?

Balance Account:

Which of these statements are true, and which are false?

1) True wealth depends far more on your attitude towards money than how much you actually have.

2) Someone with low income, properly managing money, can be much better off than a multi-millionaire who appears to have no worries.

3) Saving and investing, rather than being a deprivation, is actually the best way to earn money.

4) It is not necessary to be born into wealth to become wealthy.

5) Wealth rarely happens overnight. Most wealthy people accumulated their money over several decades.

6) Wealth is measured not only by how much you earn, but also what you keep.

7) People should plan on being able to support themselves after high school graduation, regardless of their career goals.

8) Educating yourself on financial issues, though the topic may seem unromantic, can save your relationship.

9) The time to start saving for retirement is while you're in your mid-twenties.

10) You should plan to live solely on the interest of your retirement savings, so you'll never run out of money.

Answers: All are true.

The topic of this chapter is slightly off subject, but very necessary. You have to pay for your dates somehow, and soon you will be earning your own living; your ability to do so will greatly impact the quality of your relationships. If you're constantly worrying about paying bills, either because you earn too little, or poorly manage what you have, that won't leave you much energy for reaching out to others. Even if you manage to find a partner, you will be a difficult person to live with.

The #1 thing American couples fight about is money. While it is not the primary cause for divorce, it ranks pretty high; thus, getting along financially is immensely important. It is vital you agree on monetary style, educate yourselves on the issue, and be fiscally responsible. First, how will you earn income? There are three ways; working for pay, owning a business, and investments.

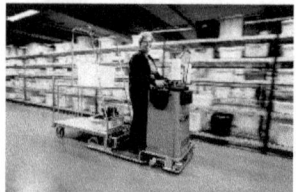

Working for pay: the greater the skills, the bigger the paycheck. Your lifestyles will depend on this, so bear in mind how you do in school affects not only you but your future spouse as well. While in high school, be sure to take courses such as auto mechanics or word processing that will enable you to earn a living wage after you graduate. If your high school does not offer such courses, you can take them at a community college or vocational school. It is best to do this during your junior year; you can take evening classes or do it over the summer. Do this even if you plan on going to college; while it's true that many people acquire their skills through additional education after high school, such an asset will help you pay bills while you study. For those who are university - bound, *DO NOT* make the mistake of assuming all you have to do to get a good job is graduate! Higher education has actually ruined many lives, with people racking up enormous student loans they can never repay and rendering them "overqualified" for whatever jobs they can do. Here is a greatly useful article describing how to avoid pitfalls and be successful: it is titled, "I Wish I'd Known This When I First Went to College!" http://sayyestolife.hubpages.com/hub/How-To-Have-A-Successful-University-Experience .

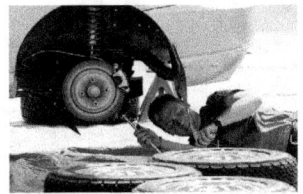

Owning a business: you can sell products, or promote your services (examples: operating a store or an auto mechanics shop). Or perhaps you were lucky to acquire some property, which you can rent out. Owning your own business is the ultimate American dream, but a mistake many people make is to look only at the gross receipts, rather than the net, which is true profit. You will need money for startup and continuing expenses, and building maintenance. Also, operating it requires a high degree of organization; you need to save money for times when sales are slow, or you're unable to work. Most businesses fail within 5 years because of mistaken ideas about its complexities. Likewise, many marriages deteriorate when couples try to operate a business together, due to the stresses involved.

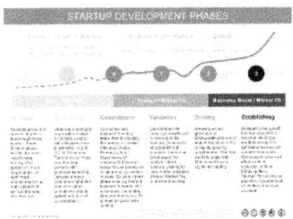

Investing: this involves lending money to companies which pay interest during the term of the loan. A basic passbook savings account is a form of investment, in which the bank is able to use the money. (There are many other forms; I will discuss these later.) The more money you have invested, the greater the amount of interest you can collect. If you're fortunate, you may have inherited a large sum of money, from which you can live off the interest. In this case, *BE CAREFUL* not to spend the principal, because your income is based on it!

Obviously, very few people are bequeathed fortunes. So how do you accumulate savings? *PAY YOURSELF FIRST!* You can put money in a jar, placing it in a savings account once a month, or shift some money from your checking account into your savings every payday. For retirement, many companies offer 401k plans; if you deduct as much as 15% of your paycheck, you'll barely notice it missing, since it is pre-taxed. Many people feel as if they're depriving themselves when they save money, rather than spend it. This belief is very destructive; the easiest way to earn money is to have it work for you. While your money is in an account accumulating interest, you're earning extra income without even thinking about it. Thus passing up frivolous purchases to save money is wise, when you consider the payoff.

Following is a list of savings and investment vehicles, where to buy them, their interest rates, and rules / regulations. Passbook savings, certificates of deposit, and money market funds pay lower interest rates but are more easily accessible, so they are best used to store emergency savings; the others, which pay 5% or higher, work better towards growing your money and providing income.

Investment Type **Passbook Savings**

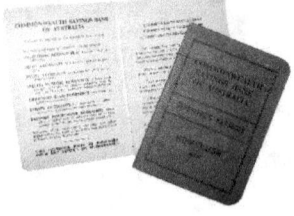

Where Available Banks, credit unions

Average Percentage Rate < 1% (credit unions offer better rates, at > 1%. Credit union membership is available based on where you work or live).

Rules Most banks require a minimum deposit, usually around $100. You can withdraw any time you want, as long as you don't dip below the minimum amount.

Investment Type **Certificate of Deposit**

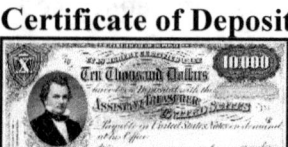

Where Available Banks, credit unions

**Average
Percentage Rate**   1% - 3%

Rules   They require a minimum deposit, usually $1000 - $5000. They must be left in for the full term chosen, which ranges from 6 months to 5 years. Penalties are levied for early withdrawal.

**Investment
Type**   **Money Market Fund**

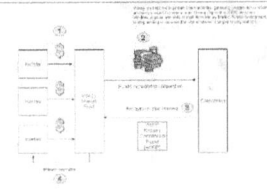

**Where
Available**   Banks, credit unions

**Average
Percentage Rate**   1% - 2%

Rules   A minimum deposit is required, usually $1000. You can withdraw from it, but are limited to a certain number of withdrawals per quarter.

**Investment
Type**   **Bonds**

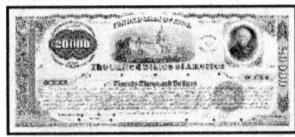

**Where
Available**   Stockbroker, financial advising company

**Average
Percentage Rate**   About 5%

Rules   These are loans to companies, which are paid upon maturity of the term. Terms can be as short as a year, or as long as 30 years. Bonds are bought in increments, usually starting as low as

151

$100. You can pay half price, getting their full value upon maturity, or you can pay full price and collect the increase at maturity. There are also coupon bonds, which pay out interest every 6 months for the full length of the term; this is good for retirement income.

Investment Type	**Stocks** 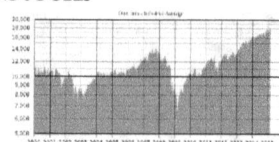
Where Available	Stockbroker, financial advising company
Average Percentage Rate	The market has averaged 11% over the past 80 years. The value can skyrocket, or the principal can lose value.
Rules	These are investments in companies. They are best bought by people who have educated themselves regarding what influences company stock value, since it is necessary to buy low and sell high.
Investment Type	**Mutual Funds** 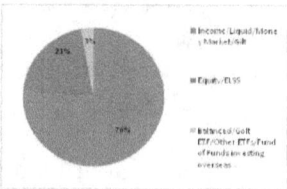
Where Available	Financial advising company, though some banks may offer them.
Average Percentage Rate	5% - 7%

Rules	This is a collection of stocks; for as little as $250, you can buy fractions of expensive shares as well as complete cheaper ones. This is the way to go for people who are not educated regarding how to choose individual stocks, since the experts managing the funds do the buying, selling and trading. Returns are lower, but also far less risky.

Investment Type

Employer Retirement Account (401k, 403b)

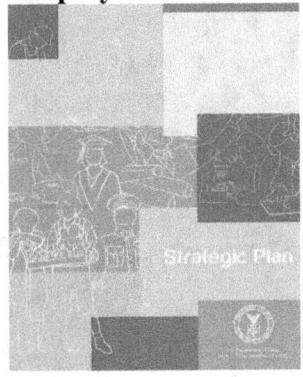

Where Available

Employers

Average Percentage Rate

5% - 7%. They are usually based on mutual funds, so the rate of return is similar.

Rules

These are opportunities for workers to save for retirement. A percentage of earnings is deducted each payday, pre-tax. Some employers match funds, providing free money to investors.

Investment Type

Individual Retirement Account (IRA)

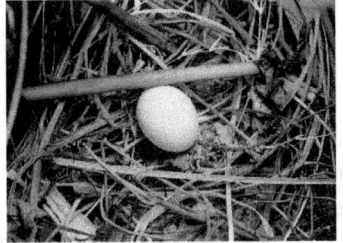

Where Available	Banks, credit unions, financial advising companies.
Average Percentage Rate	Approximately 2%; you can get higher rates if you go through a financial advising company, since they provide accounts based on stocks, bonds, and mutual funds.
Rules	You can establish your own retirement account, depositing up to $5500 per year. Contributions to a traditional account are tax-deferred, which means you don't pay tax on it until withdrawal. A Roth is not tax-deferred, but upon retirement, you withdraw from it tax free. A SEP (simplified-employee pension) is for self-employed people; it allows you to deposit up to 25% of your gross income or $52,000 per year, whichever is lesser. The SEP is tax-deferred.
Investment Type	**Annuity** 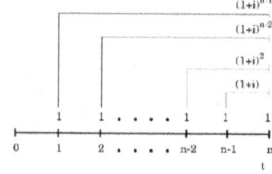
Where Available	Financial advising companies
Average Percentage Rate	Approximately 5%
Rules	This is a type of insurance. The investor puts money into the account, where it gathers interest, then upon retirement, they live off interest payments. The account must exist for a certain amount of time – 7 to 10 years, typically – before the person can withdraw from it. Also, the person must be 59½ years old before withdrawing.

154

*Special note; make sure you don't buy too late! Unscrupulous dealers have sold annuities to 70 year olds, who may not be around when it matures.

As a rule, the safer the investment, the lower the interest rate, but your money grows more slowly, and can even lag behind inflation (inflation is cost of living increase; in America, it averages 3% a year). Both of you need to decide the degree of risk you're most comfortable with. Either way, when it is time for retirement, it is best to have enough money saved in a vehicle that will enable you to live solely off the interest.

A major advantage you have to living at home is that since you have virtually no bills, you can save most of your income. Wouldn't it be fabulous if you were able to accumulate enough so that you could place your savings in a coupon bond and live off the interest, never needing to work? This is clearly not feasible for most folks; however, having a well-padded emergency fund is highly desirable. Ideally, you should amass enough to cover a year's worth of expenses, so that unexpected events, such as a major car repair or long-term unemployment, won't put you in debt. But if all else fails, have at least $1000 available so if you come up short at the end of the month, you don't have to borrow on credit cards to pay the rent or grocery bills. Also, when should you start saving for retirement? As soon as you're settled in your career, or at age 25, whichever comes first! Sure, there's social security income when you reach 67, but that's welfare, and there's no guarantee it will be around by the time you get to that age.

Once you have your income issues settled, you must work together to set up a **budget**. Again, this is *NOT* self-denial; rather, it is simply organizing your spending to avoid waste, so that you can truly afford what you need and want. While there are websites, even software, that help you, it's something you can easily do on your own. You must assess your needs. Some must be met daily, such as food and transportation. Others are monthly, like housing and utilities. Last, there are the annual / biannual expenses, such as auto insurance. First make a list, along with the price of each. Next, write your monthly income. If it is less than your outgo, you can search the list for areas to make cost adjustments.

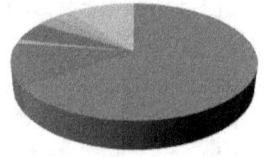

A good way to break down a budget is this way; 60% of net income should go to housing, utilities, food, clothing, and insurance. Housing alone should cost no more than 25%. The remaining 40% should go to irregular expenses (such as repairs, or vacations), long term savings, retirement, and fun money; each fund should take up approximately 10%. Optimally, you should have four savings accounts: 1) emergency funds; 2) short term goals, such as annual vacations or luxury purchases; 3) long term goals, such as down payment on a house or children's college fund; and 4) retirement savings (if you're deducting for your 401k, you will already have taken care of this).

How much can you afford for daily expenses? Simply figure out what you spend your money on every day, and the amount. Make sure it's reasonable; if you eat out on a regular basis, it's not necessary to have $20 lunches every day. It also makes more sense to brew your coffee at home, rather than driving through a stand each morning.

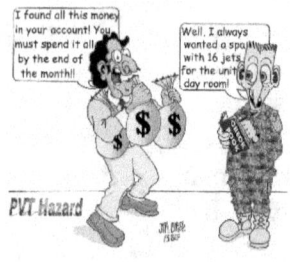

How should you spend available money on day-to day expenses? Writing checks helps you keep track of what you buy, and how much you spend on it, but that can get cumbersome. It's also impractical if you eat out a lot, since many food places don't accept checks. It's best to allow yourself a certain amount of cash each week to spend as you need, and leave the rest in your checking account, writing checks or using your debit card for purchases. *MAKE SURE YOU ALWAYS NOTIFY YOUR SPOUSE WHENEVER YOU SPEND FROM A JOINT CHECKING ACCOUNT, SO THERE ARE NO UNPLEASANT SURPRISES LATER!!!*

BORROWING / DEBT MANAGEMENT

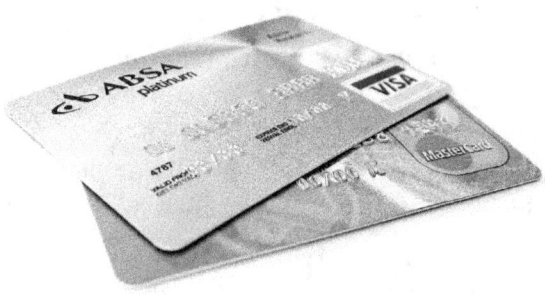

Credit cards are an absolute necessity in this day and age. One obvious reason is, they provide a quick and simple way to obtain loans. With them, you can pay for moderately expensive items, such as designer clothing or a vacation. They can also be used for cash advances. However, it is very easy to get into trouble using credit cards. Accumulating financial obligations for frivolous purchases could mean you're still paying for them long after their usefulness, so one must always count the true cost whenever deciding to take on such liabilities. Because you are charged interest on your purchases and loans, you will pay more than the ticket price; the higher the interest rate and / or the longer you take to get rid of your bill, the more the item costs. It is best to pay off credit card balances every month. If you *must* carry a balance, due to an unexpected expense such as major auto repairs, make sure your total debt does not exceed 15% of your annual income. This is called debt to income ratio (divide your annual income by your debt, and move the decimal over two places). A debt to income ratio higher than 20% will not only make your life uncomfortable, it will impact your ability to obtain a mortgage or get a low interest rate on major loans.

Horror stories of folks whose economic lives have been ruined through credit cards have frightened a lot of people away from using them altogether. You must realize, though, that there are many other reasons why they are indispensable. They are used to establish a credit rating, enabling you to rent an apartment once you move out on your own. Some employers check this before deciding to hire an applicant, since it can determine how responsible the person may be, so it can affect your ability to get a job. Also, as I stated in Chapter Four, any purchase you make online or over the phone is best done with a credit card, to protect you in case you inadvertently become a victim of fraud. Credit cards are often required to rent a car, or make hotel reservations. They can be used as a backup emergency fund if you have not yet saved enough (but save, anyway; don't rely strictly on that!). As long as you use credit cards responsibly, they can serve you very well throughout life, so there is no need to fear them.

In order to qualify for a credit card, most people have to be 21 years old; they can be as young as 18, if they're working full time. Kids still in high school can obtain one if they have their parents co-sign. This means if they run up a bill they can't pay, the parents are liable. Since this guarantees strained family relations, it is best if high schoolers practice responsibility by using pre-paid cards, so they can only "charge" as much money as is loaded on them. They can also open a checking account and use a debit card based on that. It works the same way; you can "charge" only up to the amount you have in the checking account. Special note: *DO NOT WRITE CHECKS FOR MONEY THAT IS NOT IN YOUR ACCOUNT!* This is called Passing Bad Checks. If your check bounces, most companies will require you pay for the item plus an additional fee – usually $25 - $30. If it becomes obvious you're being fraudulent with your checking account, you could be sued, or go to jail. Once it registers on your credit rating, it can be ruined big time. Potential employers may overlook an occasional lapse in judgment, or someone going through hard times, but nobody wants to hire a person who is blatantly dishonest!

For purchases that cost far more than the average person can pay cash for, such as a car or house, you can get a loan and pay by installment. Loans are available through banks, credit unions, and mortgage companies. Ideally, a person should never go into debt, but this is impractical for most, so it is vital to do this wisely. Choose an interest rate as low as you can find, and pay off the item as soon as possible. If you can afford to do so, make extra payments to erase the debt early.

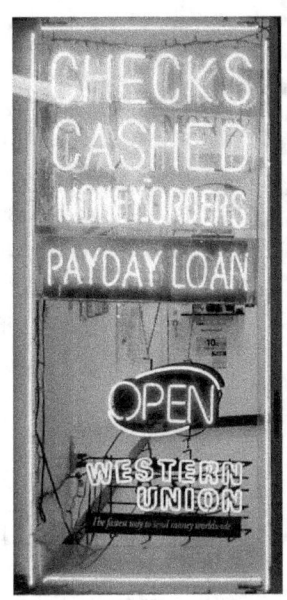

Special note: *BEWARE OF PAYDAY LOANS!!!* People who come up short before their next paycheck may be tempted go to a check-cashing place to get an advance for a set fee that seems small, but it is easy to fall behind and do this every payday; the end result is a percentage rate that ranks well into the triple digits!

Once you've worked out your personal budget, you'd be surprised at what you can afford.

Here are some additional factors to consider.

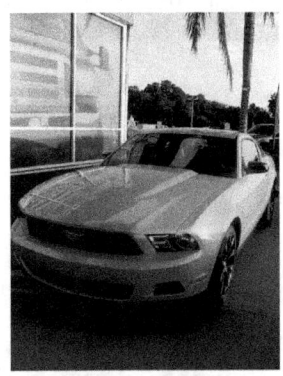

Auto insurance: Everyone who owns / drives a car needs to carry at least liability insurance. The laws against driving without insurance are *extremely* harsh. You can have your driver's license revoked and your car impounded, and be levied a hefty fine. If you get in a car accident, the other person can sue you for damages, garnishing your wages for years. You will be required to get insurance before you get your license reinstated, and the rates will be far greater than they would have been originally. Special note: *DO NOT DRINK AND DRIVE!* Getting arrested for this is a surefire way to make your rates skyrocket!

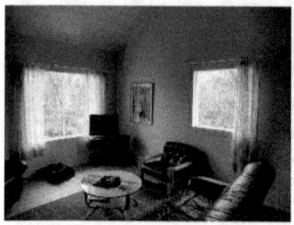

Personal (renters) insurance: if you lose your personal property in case of theft, fire, or natural disasters, this will provide you with money to replace it. It will also protect you in case you are sued. You can purchase a reasonably-priced premium through your auto insurance company. When you buy a home, homeowner's insurance covers all these, as well as protecting your house.

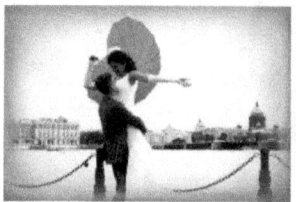

Weddings and Honeymoons: The average cost of a wedding in the US ranges from $16,000 to $86,000, depending on where the couple lives. That doesn't count the wedding gown, tuxedo, and honeymoon. Obviously, going into major debt at the start of a marriage puts unneeded stress on it; even if you have that kind of money, it's best to save it for expenses after you marry. With careful planning, weddings can be done for a few hundred dollars. Honeymoons taken in atypical locations are not only less pricey, the couple can also avoid crowds and get better customer service – and, most likely, make better memories. My favorite high school teacher's honeymoon was spent in Lassen National Park. She and her new husband were climbing the mountain when a thunderstorm blew in; at one point, lightning struck below them! Shared experiences like that can't be bought at any price.

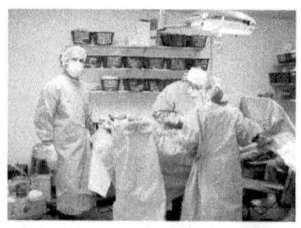

Medical / dental insurance: while a single person may (inadvisably) get along without this, you wind up with double trouble if both of you do so. This problem further increases if children are involved. You can acquire medical insurance through your workplace, or purchase it directly from the insurance company; prices vary according to the deductible, number of family members, and what procedures are covered. Make sure you're getting a real policy, rather than paying for one that will rip you off later (it is safest to go with a major company; even bare bones

160

benefits are better than nothing). People who fall below a certain income level may qualify for federally-funded Medicaid.

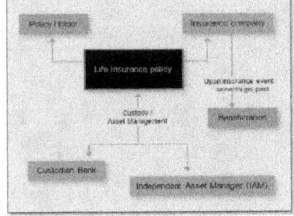

Life insurance: this takes care of your loved ones if something should happen to you. When you're on your own, if you die, your expenses cease and your debts are written off; if you have a spouse, he or she will inherit your debt, and if you have dependents, they will need your income whether or not you can provide it. So taking on life insurance is an act of love. There are two types, term, which is paid for a short while and covers only certain events, and whole life, which is a type of bank account that grows over the years and pays the survivors for the rest of their lives. They can be bought at auto insurance companies; most premiums are reasonably priced.

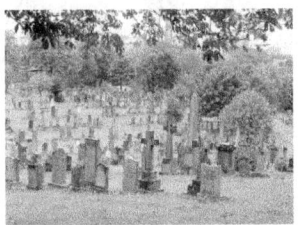

Burial insurance: many life insurance policies cover this. This pays for your funeral and burial expenses after you die. The average cost of a funeral runs from $2000 to $7000, with cremation on the cheaper end of the scale. No one likes to dwell on this subject, but worst of all would be for your loved ones to start thinking about it after experiencing the trauma of your death – so it's best to plan this early and get it over with (my favorite high school teacher and her husband did this in their early 20s).

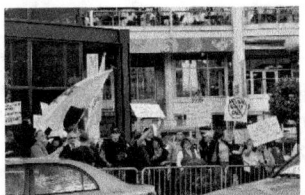

Living will: medical technology has improved the quality of life in many ways, but has also raised some new issues. Now life can be extended far beyond the body's ability to function; however, its quality is an entirely different matter. Do you want to be hooked up to a machine until you're brain dead? Do you want heroic measures taken, at any cost, to preserve your life if you were to become incapacitated? It is vital that you and your spouse discuss these issues, and get documented evidence regarding your wishes. This form is also a way to designate a Power of Attorney, someone who will speak for you and act on your behalf in the case you are unable to do so.

161

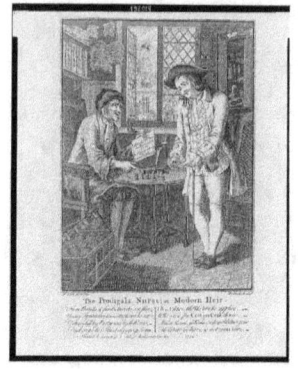

Inheritance: each state has its laws regarding who inherits money from whom; it is best if you review these laws, and make sure that is what you want. In cases of remarriage due to divorce, these laws can work against the new spouse. It may also exclude some children, and perhaps you may want to leave some of your money to other relatives or favorite charities. Be aboveboard and thorough when discussing these issues, backing them up with legal documents; you can file your own living trust online for $60 (a trust, unlike a will, avoids probate, making things much quicker and easier for your beneficiaries). As far as heirlooms are concerned, discuss who gets what well before you die, coming to an agreement, so your family isn't divided by fighting and jealousy later. Make sure the legacy you leave is a positive one!

Throughout this book, I have discussed the importance of wholesome living. Avoiding the vices of drugs and alcohol, careless living, making enemies through abuse, and greed (spending more than you earn) not only improve your quality of life but your finances as well. Regarding finances, there is one additional warning to heed:

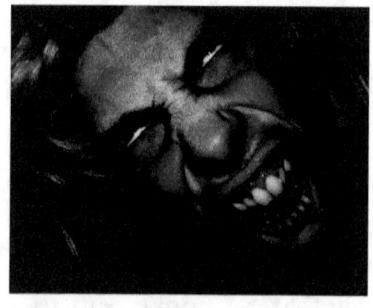

Haters and Destroyers. You may have noticed adults are reluctant to discuss how much money they make. That is because doing so makes them vulnerable to people seeking to take advantage of them. Those who earn "too little" may be made fun of for not being successful enough, or worse yet, attract shysters who lure them into investing in phony get rich quick schemes. Those who earn "too much" are often begrudged, to the point where they are subjected to outright hostility. Many appear to be popular, but their so-called friends are only using them. Winning the lottery has actually destroyed many lives, with some relatives even attempting to have the newly wealthy person murdered.

You may think a high school student working a part time minimum wage job won't have this problem, but the terms "too much" and "too little" are highly subjective. If you live in a ghetto, your peers could resent you having a job, and adults may be bitter about the fact that you have no bills to pay (some teens escaping a gang – infested neighborhood have had to go so far as to flee hundreds of miles away and take out an obituary!). In a wealthy suburb, you may encounter kids who laugh at your choices to be responsible, rather than blowing every cent on bling. In either case, people can find a way to rob you, either through violence, coercion, or identity theft. It is for these reasons you must be extremely selective with whom you discuss your salary or how much you have saved. Only people who are actively helping you in this endeavor should have that information. Such questions are intrusive and inappropriate, anyway. If anyone asks, you can respond with, "That's a rude question". You can also say, "What I have / earn is adequate" or, to a boorish adult, "I'm working towards my future, rather than assuming good luck will be handed me."

If you need a guide that will help you manage your money and create a strategy for living the life of your dreams, read my book, *Escape the Apocalypse Through Future and Financial Planning.* Currently, only the Hawaii Edition is available, but it teaches the basics which anyone can use anywhere. I will eventually publish many more editions.

In conclusion, money is a powerful tool. Ultimately, true wealth is measured not in how many fancy objects people have, but how well they have learned to manage their finances. Shown proper respect, money will serve you well and greatly improve your quality of life; educating yourself about it, exercising discipline with its usage, and being open and honest communicating with your partner is well worth the effort.

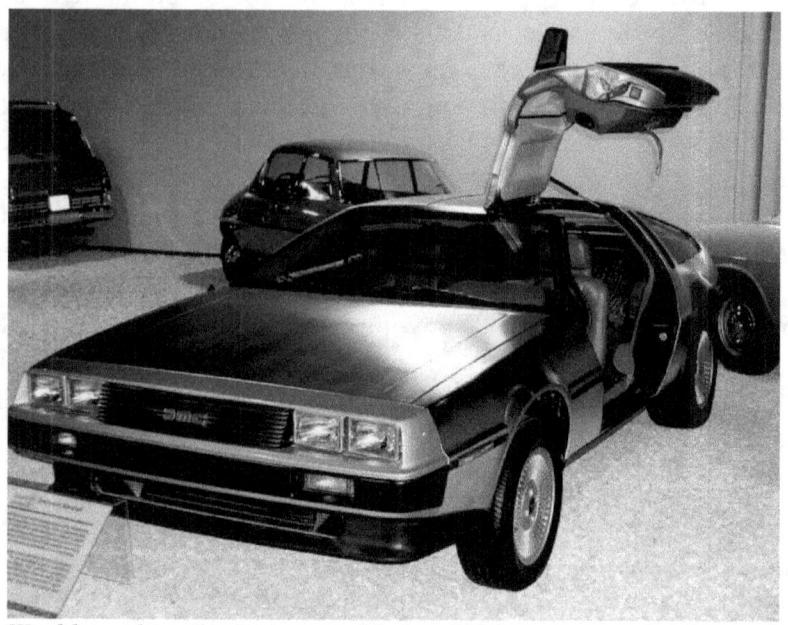

Would you drive this 24 karat gold-plated DeLorean on an LA freeway?

Settle Your Estate:

1)   Here is an activity a child of any age can do with his or her allowance.

    In the Christian Bible, Matthew 25: 14 – 30 tells a story about a master who gave 3 of his servants a certain amount of money to invest, then left on a journey. When he returned, his servants had to give account of what they did with the money given them. The first two had doubled their money, but the third didn't bother to try. That servant was punished.

    Several years ago, a Sunday School teacher gave each of her students $10 to see how they would invest it. One boy spent all his money on seeds, grew plants, and sold them at a fair. He profited over $100!

    Think of ways you can invest and increase your allowance, rather than blowing it every payday.

    Another thing; one moral given to this Bible story is that those who have much will be given more, and those who have nothing will lose even what they have. What do you suppose is meant by this moral?

2)   Junior Achievement is an organization which partners up with local businesses to educate youth about the world of employment and economics. Working with students as early as kindergarten, they teach them to operate their own companies, study investments, and give them chances to earn income. Offices are situated nearly everywhere in the US, and in many countries worldwide. Look on the web for the nearest Junior Achievement office near you. Here is their website: https://www.juniorachievement.org/web/ja-usa/home If no office is located in your area, most likely there is a subsidiary site; simply type "Junior Achievement" and your city and state in a search engine to find it. Taking part will do much to land you a good job upon graduation, whether from high school, trade school, or college.

3) Find out the cost of living in your area. These should be included:

Rent		Buying / servicing a car	
Personal (Renters) Insurance		Annual Car Registration	
Food (weekly groceries)		Annual Car Insurance	
Health Insurance		Entertainment	
Utilities		Clothing	
Commuting (gas or public transportation)		Taxes (federal as well as state)	

Now, find out the average wage of the place where you live. What jobs pay this wage? What sort of training do you need for these jobs? Can you get the training in your home town, or do you have to go elsewhere? (If you wish to relocate to another town, you can do these same exercises for that place.)

Calculate how much it would cost for you to move out on your own. These should be included: first month's rent plus deposit, enough money to turn on utilities, and furniture for your new place. You should already be working; that will serve as your credit rating. You should also have at least 1 month's worth of expenses for emergency savings in the bank, or absolute minimum $1000.

4) If you double $1 twenty times, or $1000 ten times, you will wind up with over a million dollars. Figure out how to do this

by the time you reach age 67 (you can make the age even lower, if you want to retire earlier). Hint: use the Rule of 72. Dividing 72 by your interest rate shows you how many years it will take for your money to double just by sitting in your account. Adding to it speeds up the process.

The following page contains an example of what you can do if you start with $5000, put it in a bond or mutual fund that averages a 7% return, and add $5000 to it every year. The formula is: original deposit times 1.07 = amount you'll have after one year; plus next deposit times 1.07 = amount you'll have after 2 years; etc. The deposit amounts and percentages can be adjusted according to what you wish to accomplish.

Initial Deposit	End of Year One	Year Two	Year Three	Year Four
$5,000	$10,350	$16,074.5	$22,199.72	$28,753.7
Year Five	Year Six	Year Seven	Year Eight	Year Nine
$35,766.45	$43,270.1	$51,299.01	$59,889.94	$69,082.23
Year Ten	Year Eleven	Year Twelve	Year Thirteen	Year Fourteen
$78,918	$89,442.26	$100,703.2	$112,752.4	$125,645.1
Year Fifteen	Year Sixteen	Year Seventeen	Year Eighteen	Year Nineteen
$139,440.3	$154,201.1	$169,995.2	$186,894.9	$204,977.5
Year Twenty	Year Twenty-one	Year Twenty-two	Year Twenty-three	Year Twenty-four
$224,325.9	$245,028.7	$267,180.7	$290,883.4	$316,245.2
Year Twenty-five	Year Twenty-six	Year Twenty-seven	Year Twenty-eight	Year Twenty-nine
$343,382.4	$372,419.2	$403,488.5	$436,732.7	$472,304
Year Thirty	Year Thirty-one	Year Thirty-two	Year Thirty-three	Year Thirty-four
$510,365.2	$551,090.8	$594,667.1	$641,293.8	$691,184.4
Year Thirty-five	Year Thirty-six	Year Thirty-seven	Year Thirty-eight	Year Thirty-nine
$744,567.3	$801,687	$862,805.1	$928,201.5	$998,175.6

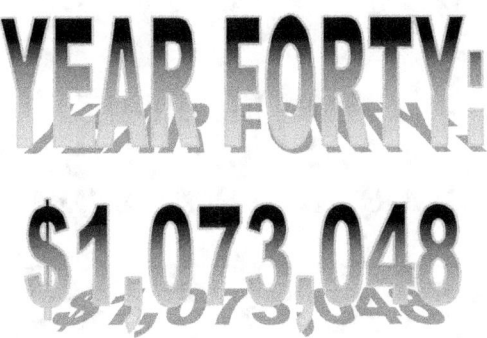

YEAR FORTY:

$1,073,048

You will have put in $205,000

Your interest will have contributed $868,048!

Another hint: One painless way to do this is to get a job that pays at least $33,334 per year, and put 15% of your pay into a 401k that averages 7%. You'll accumulate your fortune virtually unaware!

CHAPTER EIGHT

TOMORROW IS NOT PROMISED YOU, BUT…

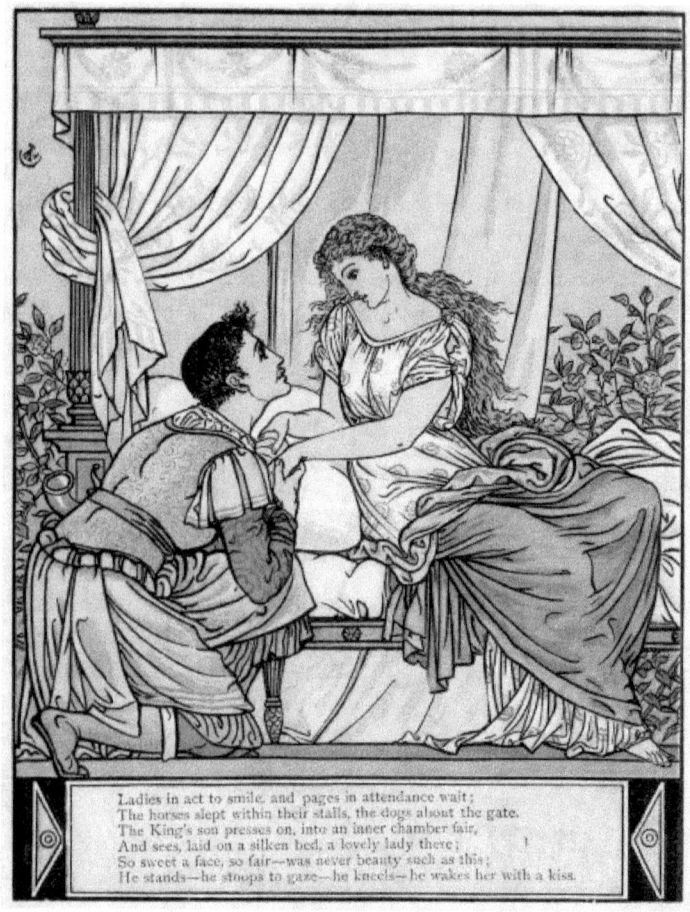

Walter Crane, Public Domain Illustration

"The road to true love will be barred by many more dangers…"
~ from *Sleeping Beauty*

Gather Intelligence:

Which of these statements are true, and which are false?

1) The American divorce rate, though among the highest in the world, varies according to region, religion, and race; therefore, knowledge and culture plays a role in the divorce rate.

2) The American divorce rate hovers around 50%.

3) What makes a marriage work is the husband and wife being truly committed and respecting each other, rather than being madly in love.

4) College educated women have a harder time getting married than those who have never attended college.

5) The highest divorce rate is in the Bible Belt South; the lowest is in the Northeast.

6) If a couple is experiencing marital problems, having a child will help hold the marriage together.

7) Whether or not marriage is better than singlehood is dependent solely on the couple.

8) Divorce is harmless if the couple has no children.

9) Each other's families should be of prime consideration when deciding to marry.

10) Living together is virtually the same as being married; the only difference is legislation and a mere piece of paper.

Answers: 1, 3, 5, 7 and 9 are true;
2, 4, 6, 8 and 10 are false.

171

So you finally meet the love of your life, and want to spend eternity with him or her. Now what?

With the divorce rate at an all-time high, people have good reason to fear marriage. While breaking up is better than being trapped in a negative, even dangerous, situation, the bottom line is, it is an aberration; a crime against nature. Divorce destroys the home of the children involved, and shreds the fabric of society. Even if there are no children, the newly single adults are almost always worse off than if they'd never wed in the first place.

In the past, society could not support single parents, so once you married, that was *IT* - even in cases of abuse. So both parties were carefully coached and counseled; in some societies, marriages were even arranged by the parents or village matchmaker! In America today, family is often not even considered; yet, ultimately, it is really them you are marrying, not just your spouse. Even if they're not around, they made your partner what he or she is today, so they still have influence.

However, there is good news on the subject. Divorce is not nearly as prevalent as people have been led to believe. The American 50% rate is based on the number of marriages and divorces in any given year. A more accurate calculation is to count how many people have ever been divorced; in this case, it ranks closer to 25%. This statistic also varies according to region (highest in the South, lowest in the Northeast), race (highest African American, lowest Asian), and religion (highest among non-denominational Christians, lowest among atheists. The statistics regarding religion may come as a surprise to some; the explanation is, conservative Christian groups are often reluctant to discuss sexual matters, maintaining a strict abstinence policy among singles while pressuring them to marry, whereas atheists don't exert such pressure, and are more hard-core realistic about situations, openly addressing and discussing them). Evidently, education and culture play major roles in determining the strength and quality of a union.

Let's face it; matrimony is best when it's done right the first time. So how can you avoid divorce? Bear in mind not everyone is suitable for nuptial ties; to succeed, you need certain traits that make you easy to live with. Being a good partner is every bit as important as finding one.

Following are the most important traits to possess for you to be an ideal partner.

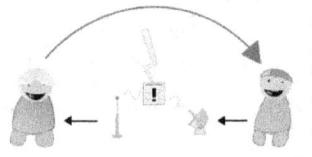 **Good communication skills / openness.** The number one reason for divorce is constant conflict. Often people wed for the wrong reasons; to avoid loneliness, gain status, "everyone else" is getting married or, at their age, they feel tremendous social pressure to do so. A teenager may be desperate to escape a negative home situation; others unrealistically expect marriage will save them in some way (a common belief among addicts). Perhaps they see faults in their partner, but they feel they invested too much time in the relationship, or they're convinced they won't find anyone else. Or they may be totally enamored, causing them to rush to the altar – only to find out later, when emotions have cooled, that they don't really know one another. A long time ago, I heard a story about a couple who couldn't keep their hands off each other, so they wanted to hurry up and marry before they committed fornication. The minister agreed to do so, on the condition that they were to be strictly chaperoned for a week; they were to not so much as hold hands. Reluctantly, they went along. At the end of the week, the woman went into the minister's office – alone. "Forget the wedding; he's the most boring person on Earth!" she exclaimed.

It is critical to make clear who you truly are, what you need, and your personal aspirations. You must also be able to respect your partner; this is more important than love, which comes and goes (lack of respect is guaranteed to kill it). Also, always let them know what you're thinking; don't assume he or she can read your mind. This helps you grow together as well; everyone changes over time, and you don't want to turn into strangers. Good communication skills are key!

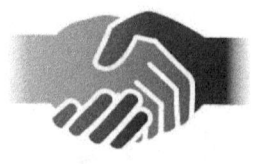 **Honesty/Trustworthiness**. When it comes to important relationships of any kind, hypocrites and compulsive liars need not apply. Nobody wants to be saddled with someone they can't believe or trust. You should have the quality of character to know the difference between right and wrong, and follow it; don't say or do anything that will make your partner regret choosing you.

Stories abound of people who put on all sorts of acts to get someone, only to reveal their true colors afterwards. For instance, a guy may say he's in love with a girl he just started dating, but his real purpose is to get her to have sex with him. Or a girl may put on an act to get a guy, saying she enjoys the same things he does, only to revert to her real self and try to change him once they're in an exclusive relationship. Either one may be seeing someone else; they reassure their partner they broke up, yet the affair continues. It may even go as far as a guy calling his girlfriend for a date, not showing up, and constantly calling to reassure her he'll be there in awhile, when in reality he out with someone else. Or a girl may tell her boyfriend she is pregnant with his baby, when either she isn't, or she is but someone else is the father. The list is endless. So how do you avoid such a person? You need to be an honest, trustworthy person yourself. Equally important, the first time you catch your partner in a lie, break it off immediately. They will definitely do it again, and once you're dependent on them, it will only get worse.

In addition, do not betray your partner's trust. If he or she tells you something that is to be kept confidential, *RESPECT THAT*. Also, whenever you tell them something that you want to keep a secret, make that clear; they should respect your wishes too.

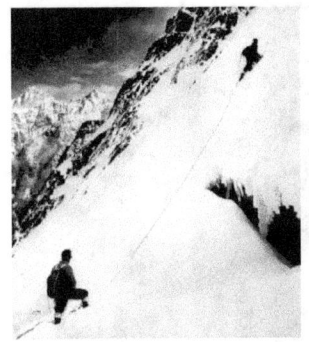

Ability to Trust. A chronically suspicious person is a major drain. If you made a wise choice, there is no need for obsessive jealousy. People who are constantly wary tend to have low self-esteem, making them. more likely to resort to manipulative tactics or be flat-out abusive. If you have this trait, get counselling so you don't drive away your potential soul mate

C *om* **passion**

Empathy / compassion. Once you're in a relationship, it's no longer all about you. Everything you do, every decision you make, you need to consider how this affects your partner. The ability to share is one of the most vital traits to maintaining a relationship.

Patience / Tolerance.

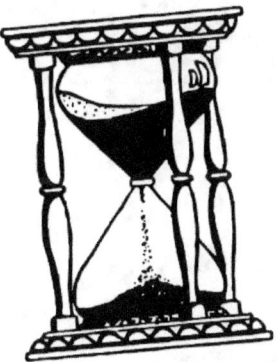

Sense of humor.

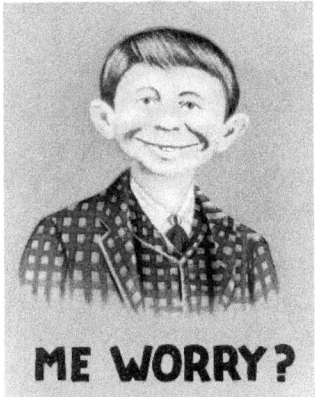

Not everyone does things at the same pace you do. Likewise, you don't do things at the same pace others do. When you're joined with someone, you need to take these factors into consideration.

The more you can see the good in a negative situation, and even make light of it, the more people will want to be around you and the easier it will be to live with you.

175

Cleanliness/self-maintenance. When you're by yourself, your personal habits are no one's business but your own, but when you share a living space, it's definitely your partner's issue. It is extremely important to show the same consideration, if not greater, as you would show to a roommate.

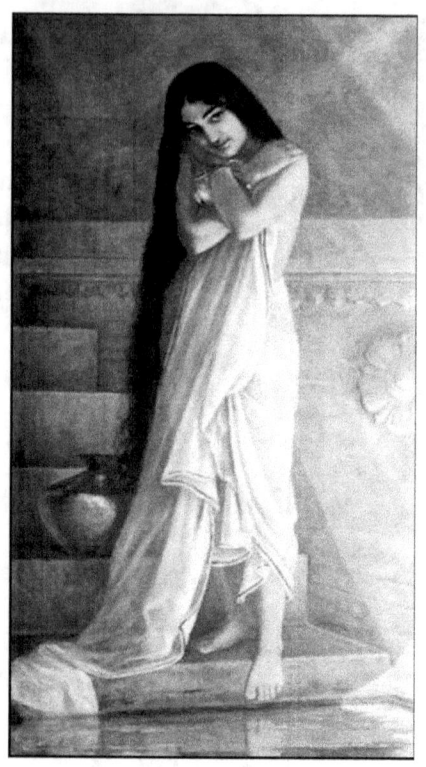

Adaptability.

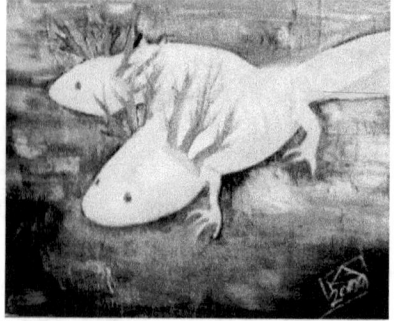

You need to know how to compromise on issues without compromising yourself.

Strong Sense of Appreciation.

Focusing on your partner's best traits and refraining from nagging regarding the negative ones will go far to keep love alive for both of you.

Likewise, there are personality traits that are practically guaranteed to destroy a relationship. Here I list the ones to be avoided / overcome at all costs.

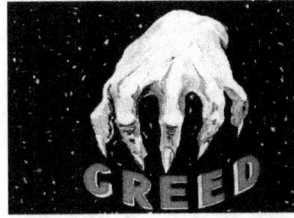

Selfishness. Marriage is a partnership; that means not only you share everything, but each decision you make, you *must* consider the other person. It's not all about you anymore. If you want the world to revolve around you, stay single.

Infidelity. If you love variety, either stay single or marry someone who loves variety too. Most people see marriage as an exclusive partnership, and no one wants to be cheated on. Besides, that kind of lifestyle carries the risks of diseases and unwanted pregnancy.

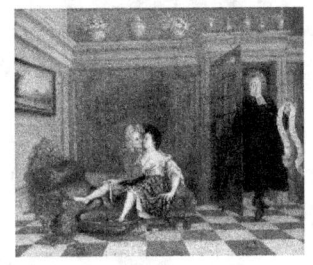

Special note; *DO NOT* casually discuss your sex life! With the exception of a licensed sex therapist, that subject is to be exclusive, strictly between you and your partner. One man told me he wondered why his wife's friends kept coming on to him; it turned out she was bragging to them about how good he was in bed!

Violent temper.

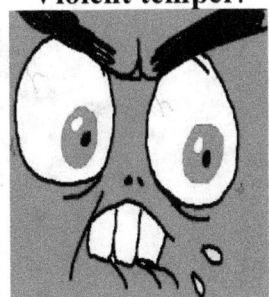

No one likes to be on the receiving end of outbursts. Also, since someone in the midst of rage isn't thinking clearly, they are more likely to say or do something they'll regret later.

Manipulating nature.

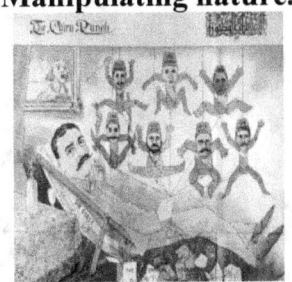

No one enjoys being manipulated. If you want something, state it openly, making your intentions clear. Needing to be underhanded about your request is a sign something is wrong with it.

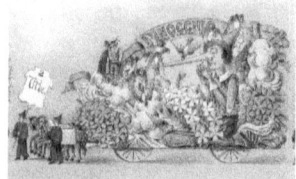

Deceptiveness. Nothing destroys relationships faster than lack of trust. Any time you're tempted to deceive your partner, ask yourself how you'd feel if he or she did it to you.

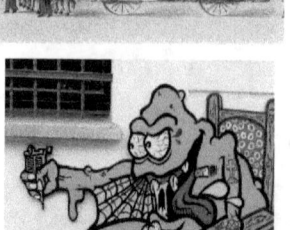

Lack of trust / jealousy. On the other hand, you should be able to trust your partner. If they're good enough for you to choose, they should be worth giving the benefit of the doubt. Excessively jealous people are extremely hard to live with. Their jealousy is usually a reflection of their own poor self - esteem rather than the trustworthiness of their partner, and such a person may even be an abuser (does this describe you?).

Substance abuse.

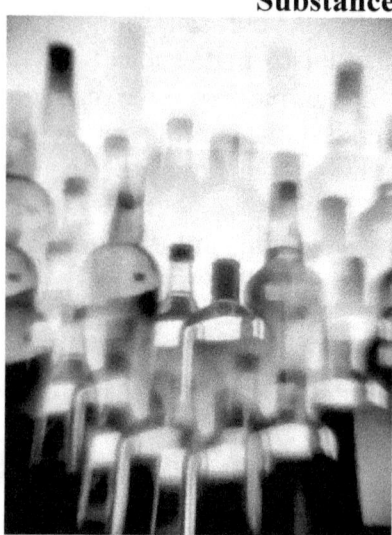

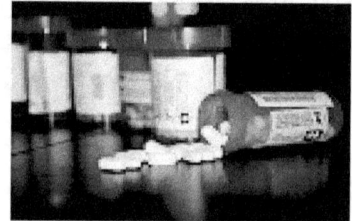

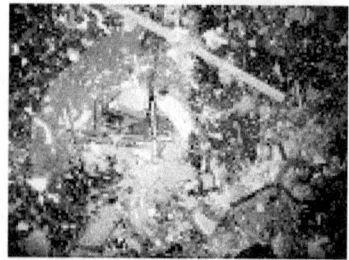

Addictions are expensive, destroy one's character, and ruin quality of life. Even as a single person, it's seldom just your business; when you have a partner, it has a tremendous effect on that person. Ask yourself, "Would I want to put up with this behavior in someone else?" If the answer is no, do whatever is necessary to overcome it. (If the answer is yes, marry someone with your same bad habits!) Besides, drugs and excessive alcohol ruin things in the bedroom.

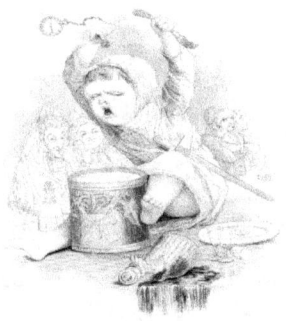

Immaturity. Marriage is for adults who are able to take care of themselves, any children they have, and appropriately deal with whatever issues come up. Sure, some societies marry off girls barely in their teens but take a good look at how oppressive they are. Is that how you want your home to be? (Women; would you marry a 13 year old boy?)

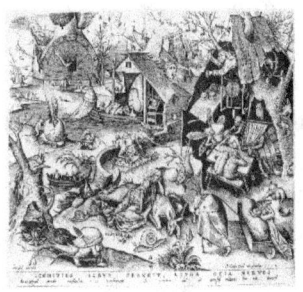

Laziness. Some people enter a partnership for a free ride. Not only is this is flat-out dishonest, it is also foolish, since it can backfire if they get dumped and wind up stranded. I know a case where a man who was a university senior married a nurse from a wealthy family. Two months before graduating with a Computer Science degree, he dropped out and lived off his wife's income. He proved to be a lousy house husband; their place was messy, and he was haphazard about taking their two children to school. When he became physically abusive, that was the last straw; her parents stepped in and put a stop to it. They helped her file for divorce, and he ultimately wound up homeless.

Pull your weight in the relationship! Focusing on what you have to offer, rather than dwelling on what you can get out of it, is a major ingredient to success.

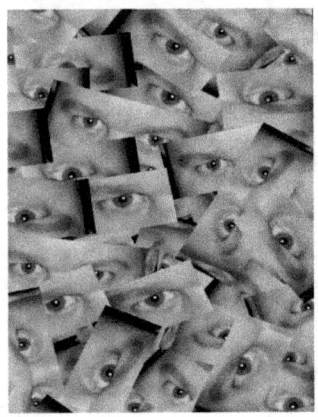

Antisocial personality. When you partner up with someone, you're also involved with their family and friends. Ideally, you should like each other's associates, since they are a reflection of that person; disliking them says negative things about the quality of the relationship. Agree on how often to visit, and allow your companion free time to hang out with them. Isolating your partner is the height of unfairness, and also a common tactic for abusers. Likewise,

179

remember your personal community, as it's only a matter of time before you need them.

Once you have developed these virtues and freed yourself of the indicated vices, you can look for a partner who has done the same. After finding him or her, you need to make sure the two of you are compatible. Here is a list of what to discuss with your potential mate – *BEFORE* marriage.

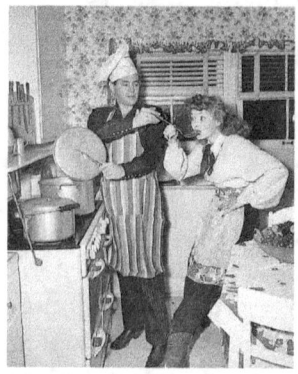

Marital roles. In previous generations, societal norms determined who did what; the husband provided financially and did the roofing and yardwork while the wife maintained the inside of the home and handled most of the childrearing tasks. Nowadays, with people marrying later, women are more likely to have careers and men need to do their own cooking and laundry. This can lead to conflict when after the wedding the wife wants to keep working, and the husband assumes she will do all the household chores and take care of the kids anyway. Since this is a major reason the divorce rate has skyrocketed over the past half century, it is of extreme importance the two of you fully discuss the matter and decide which roles you will take on. Balance in the relationship is absolutely necessary; the woman needs to contribute financially, while the man shares in the housework and parenting.

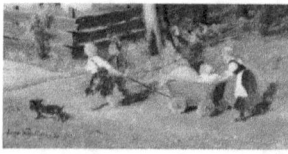

Children. This is one area where your partner's family, as well as your own, has huge influence. Sure, people can always attend parenting classes, but ultimately the way you were raised determines your attitudes towards children, including their ages and genders. It is extremely vital to agree on how many you want, how to raise them, and how involved with your respective relatives they will be. Both partners should be parents. If there is a conflict where you have to choose between your spouse and your children, you spouse should have priority; this prevents the children from playing divide-and-conquer games, plus you will still have to deal with each other after they have grown up and left home.

Also, bear in mind that human nature has a role; people do tend to play favorites, depending on the child's gender, looks, personality, and circumstances of birth. (Regarding looks, here's advice from my favorite high school teacher; "Never criticize your children's physical features, because they got them from you.")

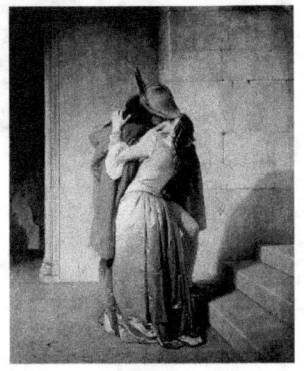

Sexual compatibility. Sex is a very important part of marriage. In the past, premarital sex was a blatant *NO* because few methods of birth control were available, and even fewer people knew about them. If after the vows were exchanged, the erotic quality was lousy or nonexistent, the couple just lived with it, or they had affairs and dealt with the consequences (out - of – wedlock births, diseases, etc.). Since so many options exist today, it is feasible to "test drive the car before buying" – however, couples must consider many factors. Having sex too soon in the relationship tends to stunt its growth and cloud judgment. In America and Great Britain, divorce statistics are slightly higher among those who cohabited before wedlock; however, in Germany and France, they are actually lower. Either way, it is best to avoid casual flings, since they produce few benefits and many risks, some of which are can either kill you or negatively affect your life forever. Whether or not you decide to abstain until marriage, the best bet is to wait until your relationship is fully mature before having sex.

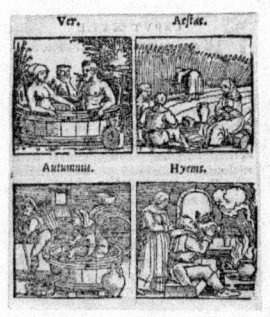

Living styles. The two of you should have similar goals in life; the more you have in common with your partner, and can agree on basics, the easier adjusting to marriage will be. Marry someone with your intelligence level, and discuss how you will deal with unforeseen difficulties, such as a job loss, long distance move, major illness, or a child with disabilities. Be of the same mind on fundamentals like politics, religion, and whatever else is important to you. However, show consideration regarding your differences. If your partner likes something you're unfamiliar with, perhaps you can learn something, expanding your horizons. You can teach your partner new things as well. As much as possible, do everything together, including grocery shopping and going to the hardware store. Have regular dates with each other. Vacation and have new experiences together.

How to manage finances. Because the #1 thing American couples fight about is money, it is important you agree on financial style and educate yourselves on this issue.

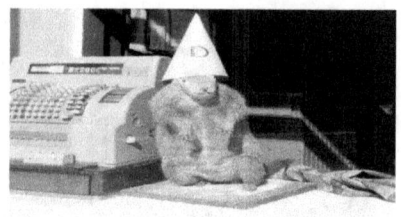

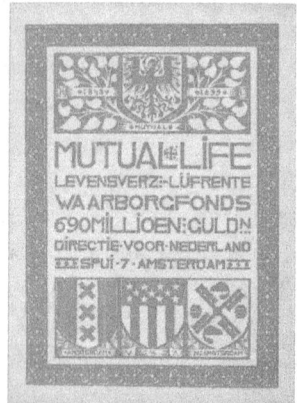

Medical / death / life insurance / living will / inheritance decisions. These topics, though far from glamorous, are *EXTREMELY* important. Saddling your partner with an enormous load of bills, or springing a nasty surprise on your family after you die, is one of the worst things you can do. Be aboveboard and thorough when discussing these issues, backing them up with legal documents. Should a crisis arise, you'll both thank each other later! (I have already discussed this subject in Chapter Seven.)

DEALING WITH EACH OTHER'S RELATIVES

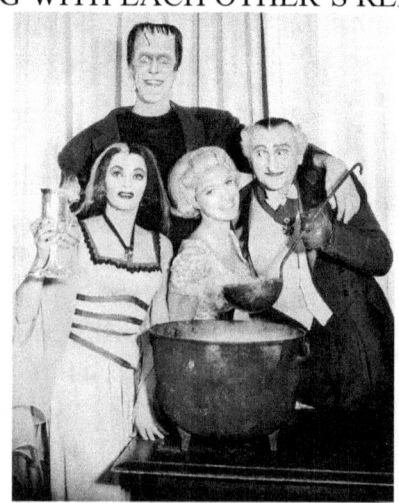

The Munsters

"Take a good look at the family - they're the ones you're really marrying!" That's the advice given to me by one of my high school teachers. Though in laws are notorious for presenting significant problems, they can actually be a major asset. If you grew up in a dysfunctional home, marriage could be an opportunity for you to acquire the ideal parents you never had.

It is extremely important to treat each other's families with respect. As much as possible, make best friends with your spouse's parents – they can't be too awful, since they raised your spouse! However, since this is easier said than done, here are some guidelines towards this end.

First, discuss the roles, and the degree of involvement, each set of parents will have in your lives. Assume *NOTHING!* Set boundaries regarding visits, being with grandchildren, helping out, giving advice, etc. Be firm with these, even if it means screening phone calls and refusing to offer duplicate keys if they don't abide by your wishes.

Do not discuss relationship conflicts with your parents. Your marriage should be exclusive, just the two of you; no one should be allowed to interfere, since if you're both adult enough to marry, you should be expected to handle your own situations. Besides complaining can give them a negative view of your spouse, especially if you don't tell them how you resolved the issue. If you can't deal with the matter yourselves, seek professional counseling.

Any troubles you have with your in-laws should be handled by your spouse. Likewise, you should be the one who talks with your parents if they have problems with your partner. As much as possible, avoid making them choose between you and their parents.

Avoid comparing your spouse to your parent. Phrases like, "My mother / father always did it this way" is a sign of immaturity, indicating perhaps you should have stayed home instead of marrying and setting up your own household.

Now, for the ultimate complication; there may be some members of either clan who are downright toxic. Perhaps they are criminals, molesters, or prone to random violence. Maybe they're none of the above, but are flat out hell bent on destroying your relationship. You must agree to not inflict these people on your spouse, even if they are your parents. Though the first people in both your lives were family, your marriage should be even more important; anyone detrimental to it should be omitted. Correspondingly, if your partner forces you to associate with relatives that abuse you, it would be wise to not marry, since you can expect far worse after the wedding (refer to my high school teacher's advice! Incidentally, she and her husband tried to resolve the issue by moving away, but ultimately they divorced).

SOME FINAL FACTORS TO CONSIDER

How long should you court before marrying? Since anyone can hide faults and fool someone over the short term, it is important to do so long enough to truly know each other. A good time frame is 2- 3 years; you should be able to see your future spouse in a wide variety of situations in that period. People from dysfunctional backgrounds should date longer, to make sure they have resolved their issues rather than repeating them.

How old should you be when you marry? Most Americans state the ideal age around 25, give or take a couple years, since at that age they'll most likely be finished with their education, fairly well established in their careers, and know what they want out of life. However, the most important factors are the couple's maturity. They should be self-sufficient and able to conduct themselves, reason, and problem solve as adults. Some people can do that at 18; others still have not achieved it at 40.

Can you accept your lover exactly as he or she is? So often, people try to change their spouse, but it rarely works – even when it does, the results are often even more disastrous. After all, why are you trying to revise your mate? If your partner is an addict, perhaps you are co-dependent, in which case the relationship would fall apart if the addiction were overcome. Or perhaps you are the sort of character who is always trying to transform others, and thus is never satisfied. As for the one you are trying to "rehabilitate", realize that their particular neurosis has worked for them all their lives, and therefore it is highly unlikely they will give it up for anyone, including you. They may pretend to do so until marriage, but afterwards they'll most likely revert right back to their old habits. The best bet is to decide whether or not you can live with their faults; if you can't, move on.

As you can see, making a marriage work takes much careful planning, and there's a lot to consider. You can fall in love with all types of people, but quality of character - yours as well as the other person's - is what determines whether or not it will succeed. In summary, remember:

1) <u>Marriage is a partnership, not a solo venture.</u> Every decision you make, every habit you have, affects your spouse. Being the right person is every bit as important as choosing the ideal partner. *Always* consider that!

2) <u>A generous, forgiving nature is vital.</u> Focus on your partner's positive traits, compliment regularly, and make them feel important. Don't sweat the petty things (pet the sweaty things instead). Also, a sense of humor goes a long way in soothing rough situations.

3) <u>Most important of all, remember the whole is greater than the sum of its parts.</u> When you marry, you give up some of the benefits of singlehood; however, you gain the advantages marriage offers. Whether or not one state is better than the other depends on what the couple makes of it. Before marrying, be sure you can agree on your differences, because you're guaranteed to have some; seek therapy if you need it. Ultimately, success depends on the determination of both partners; "Divorce" is a word that should never be part of your vocabulary

Following these precepts may not guarantee eternal bliss – after all, life itself is a gamble – but careful thinking and planning will do much to help you avoid pitfalls, and deal with whatever curve balls are thrown your way. A successful marriage is not a stroke of luck – it is an achievement.

185

Best wishes on your journey!

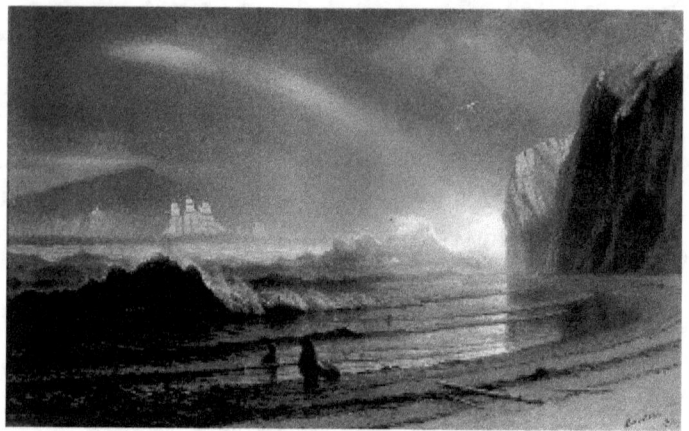

Proposal:

1) Write a letter to your future spouse; this template can give you some ideas.

What does marriage mean to you?

What do you want out of life and marriage?

Why, out of all your options, did you choose that person?

What do you have to offer your future spouse? How will you treat them? How do you want them to treat you?

Explain why that person should want you for a spouse.

Explain, in detail, your plans for your future together (where you will live, how many kids, unglamorous financial arrangements, etc.).

End the letter by saying you look forward to meeting this person (or marrying them, if you've already met them).

2. If you have someone in mind you want to marry, fill out the character profile worksheet from Chapter One about the person, and have him or her do the same about you. Compare and discuss your answers. Here is the link: http://imaginingsofacreativewriter. blogspot.com/2012/05/character-profile-sheet.html

Though it is for developing characters for novels, you two will be creating your own story together. Who knows – perhaps it will turn into the next Great American Novel!

REFERENCES

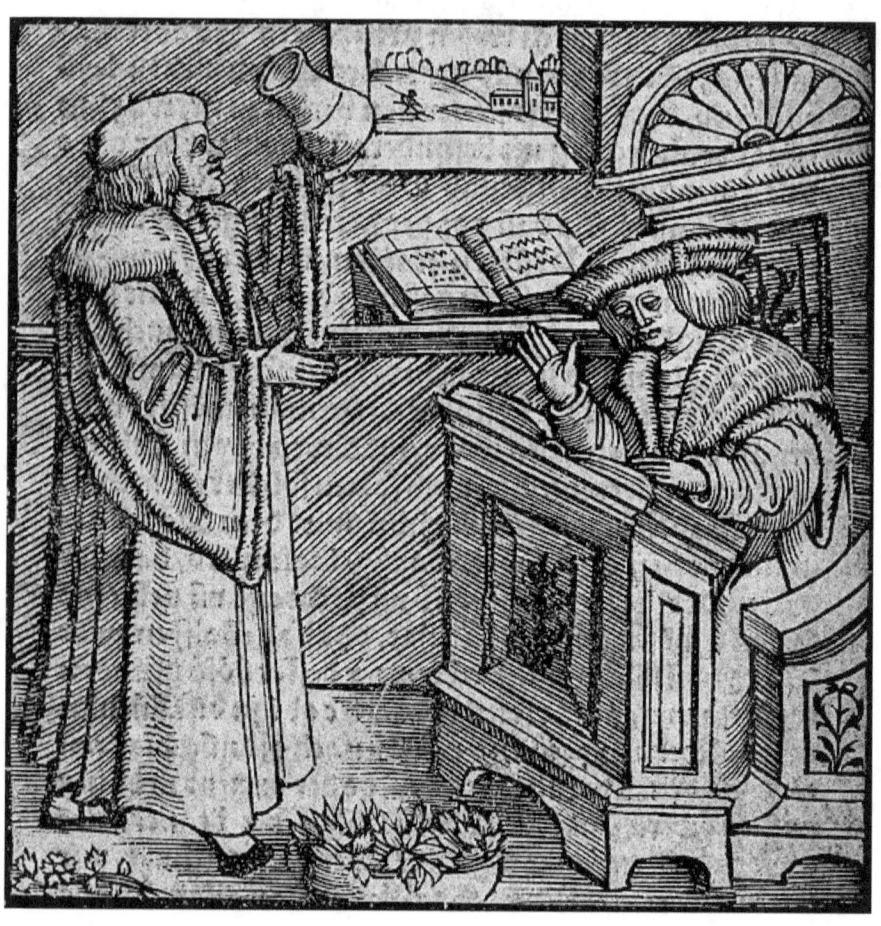

Title Page Illustration

By Gustave Doré, Public Domain,
https://commons.wikimedia.org/w/index.php?curid=678356

Table of Contents Illustration

"Stanford University Arches of Main Quad" by Fred Hsu
(Wikipedia:User:Fredhsu on en.wikipedia) - Photo taken and
uploaded by user. Licensed under CC BY-SA 3.0 via
Wikimedia Commons -
https://commons.wikimedia.org/wiki/File:Stanford_Universit
y_Arches_of_Main_Quad.jpg#/media/File:Stanford_Universi
ty_Arches_of_Main_Quad.jpg

Drop Cap Graphics

http://www.clipshrine.com/

Introduction Illustration

https://commons.wikimedia.org/wiki/File:1880_Pierre_Auguste_
Cot_-_The_Storm.jpg

Chapter One: Yes, You Can Be an Alpha Male / Female!

Patterson, James and Kim, Peter. *The Day America Told the
Truth*. Prentice Hall Trade. 1991. Print.

http://hellobeautiful.com/2012/06/01/what-women-look-for-in-
men/

http://magazine.foxnews.com/love/top-10-qualities-men-are-
secretly-looking-women

https://answers.yahoo.com/question/index?qid=20110509234046
AA1jP4A

https://answers.yahoo.com/question/index?qid=20110509234321
AANnROo

http://www.askmen.com/dating/curtsmith_100/137_dating_advic
e_a.html

http://www.chadhowsefitness.com/blog/2012/11/25-
characteristics-of-an-alpha-male/

http://www.wikihow.com/Be-the-Alpha-Female

http://datingfortodaysman.com/2011/03/alpha-female-
characteristics/

http://www.drjamesdobson.org/Solid-
Answers/Answers?a=ff773023-2693-410d-b9e1-
662f6985be4e

http://isreview.org/issue/72/are-men-really-better-athletes

http://www.lazyrunner.com/men-versus-women

http://longevity.about.com/od/wholiveslongest/f/men-women-
aging.htm

http://consumer.healthday.com/senior-citizen-information-
31/misc-aging-news-10/mouth-area-wrinkles-more-in-
women-than-men-634104.html

Illustrations

"Rome murales 03" by Nicholas Gemini - Own work. Licensed under CC BY-SA 3.0 via Wikimedia Commons – https://commons.wikimedia.org/wiki/File:Rome_murales_03. JPG#/media/File:Rome_murales_03.JPG

http://commons.wikimedia.org/wiki/File:Connecticut_ComiC ONN_Superhero_Mascot..jpg

https://commons.wikimedia.org/wiki/File:Shiko.jpg

https://commons.wikimedia.org/wiki/File:RIAN_archive_10347 9_Soviet_weight-lifter_Viktor_Mazin_during_the_XXII_Olympic_Games.jpg

https://commons.wikimedia.org/wiki/File:Gymnast_jumping_on _beam.jpg

https://commons.wikimedia.org/wiki/File:Life_Expectancy_U.S. _Trends_(Alt).png

"Ushuaia recreacion penal lou" by Lourdes Cardenal - Own work. Licensed under GFDL via Wikimedia Commons - http://commons.wikimedia.org/wiki/File:Ushuaia_recreacion _penal_lou.JPG#/media/File:Ushuaia_recreacion_penal_lou.J PG

https://commons.wikimedia.org/wiki/File:Flame_002.png

https://commons.wikimedia.org/wiki/File:An_old_woman_with_ a_crumpled_face,_wearing_elaborate_costume_Wellcome_V 0009448ER.jpg

https://commons.wikimedia.org/wiki/File:An_old_woman_with_ a_crumpled_face,_wearing_elaborate_costume_Wellcome_V 0009448ER.jpg

191

http://commons.wikimedia.org/wiki/File:Portugalete_-_Graffiti_1.jpg

https://commons.wikimedia.org/wiki/File:Betty_Boop_patent_fig1.jpg

"Ideology Icon". Licensed under Public Domain via Wikimedia Commons - http://commons.wikimedia.org/wiki/File:Ideology_Icon.png#/media/File:Ideology_Icon.png

https://commons.wikimedia.org/wiki/File:Man_and_woman_holding_baloons.svg
https://commons.wikimedia.org/w/index.php?curid=19757623

Chapter Two: All the Good Ones are Taken – *Really?*

http://www.askmen.com/top_10/dating/top-10-new-places-to-meet-women.html

http://www.complex.com/city-guide/2013/09/20-places-to-meet-women-that-arent-bars/chuck-e-cheese-or-other-child-centric-spot

http://allwomenstalk.com/10-best-places-to-meet-eligible-men

http://en.wikipedia.org/wiki/Teen_online_dating

http://www.huffingtonpost.com/claire-mccarthy-md/online-dating-for-teens_b_3682486.html

http://www.boardgamecapital.com/smart-ass-rules.htm

http://www.familyandpartygames.com/loadedquestions.html

http://theboardgamenut.blogspot.com/2009/12/say-anything.html

http://ehealthmd.com/content/problems-caused-alcohol

http://money.usnews.com/money/personal-finance/articles/2015/06/02/the-etiquette-of-paying-for-dates-today

http://www.eharmony.com/dating-advice/dating-advice-for-you/going-dutch-on-a-date-good-idea/#.VkVYAGfJCM8

http://www.mensfitness.com/women/dating-advice/its-2014-who-should-pay-date

http://www.huffingtonpost.com/2015/06/29/paying-on-the-first-date_n_7673180.html

http://www.niaaa.nih.gov/alcohol-health/special-populations-co-occurring-disorders/underage-drinking

Illustrations

https://commons.wikimedia.org/wiki/File:The_Frog_Prince_and_Other_Stories-illus007s.jpg

"CrescentMoon2" by Jessmcintyre - Own work. Licensed under CC BY-SA 3.0 via Wikimedia Commons - https://commons.wikimedia. org/wiki/File:CrescentMoon2.JPG#/media/File:CrescentMoon2.JPG

https://commons.wikimedia.org/wiki/File:New_Zealand_-Dance_class_-_9514.jpg

"Talwalkars launched Zumba Fitness Programme in India, Neha Dhupia" by http://www.bollywoodhungama.com - http://www.bollywoodhungama.com/more/photos/view/stills/parties-and-events/id/1452034. Licensed under CC BY 3.0 via Wikimedia Commons - https://commons.wikimedia.org/wiki/File:Talwalkars_launched_Zumba_Fitness_Programme

https://commons.wikimedia.org/wiki/File:2006_Pro_Bowl_tackle.jpg#/media/File:2006_Pro_Bowl_tackle.jpg

https://commons.wikimedia.org/wiki/File:Plucked_string_instruments_(2)_Mandolin,_Lute,_Portuguese_string_ensemble,_Portuguese_guitar_-_Soinuenea.jpg

https://commons.wikimedia.org/wiki/File:Auto_Repair_shop.jpg

https://commons.wikimedia.org/wiki/File:Computer-aj_aj_ashton_01.svg

https://commons.wikimedia.org/wiki/File:Leonid_Meteor_Storm_1833.jpg

https://commons.wikimedia.org/wiki/File:Escalade_amellago.jpg

https://commons.wikimedia.org/wiki/File:Skateboard_park,_Marble_Falls,_TX_IMG_1976.JPG

https://commons.wikimedia.org/wiki/File:420_Class_Dinghies_with_spinnakers.jpg

https://commons.wikimedia.org/wiki/File:Golf_twilight_golf.jpg

https://commons.wikimedia.org/wiki/File:Wien_Cafe_Central_2004.jpg

https://commons.wikimedia.org/wiki/File:BHS-Cafeteria.jpg

"Luke Witkowski 2015-04-11" by Gspeed0689 - Own work. Licensed under CC BY 4.0 via Wikimedia Commons - https://commons.wikimedia.org/wiki/File:Luke_Witkowski_2015-04-11.jpg#/media/File:Luke_Witkowski_2015-04-11.jpg

"Cain USA Nebelhorn 2013". Licensed under CC BY-SA 3.0 via Wikimedia Commons -

https://commons.wikimedia.org/wiki/File:Cain_USA_Nebelh
orn_2013.JPG#/media/File:Cain_USA_Nebelhorn_2013.JPG

https://commons.wikimedia.org/wiki/File:Earthjustice_Logo.jpg

"Obama family performing community service 1-09" by
Executive Office of the President - Source. Licensed under
Public Domain via Wikimedia Commons -
https://commons.wikimedia.org/wiki/File:Obama_family_per
forming_community_service_1-
09.jpg#/media/File:Obama_family_performing_community_
service_1-09.jpg

https://commons.wikimedia.org/wiki/File:Churchangle.jpg

By Liface at the English language Wikipedia, CC BY-SA 3.0,
https://commons.wikimedia.org/w/index.php?curid=2686033

https://commons.wikimedia.org/wiki/File:Le_doigt_magique_ou
_le_magnetisme_animal%27_Wellcome_L0000477EB.jpg

"Pharyngeal flap procedures3" by The original uploader was
Felsir at English Wikipedia - Transferred from en.wikipedia
to Commons.. Licensed under CC BY-SA 3.0 via Wikimedia
Commons - https://commons.wikimedia.org/wiki/
File:Pharyngeal_flap_procedures3.gif#/media/File:Pharyngea
l_flap_procedures3.gif

"Presa de decissions" by Martorell - Self-published work by
Martorell. Licensed under CC BY-SA 3.0 via Wikimedia
Commons - https://commons.wikimedia.
org/wiki/File:Presa_de_decissions.png#/media/File:Presa_de
_decissions.png

https://commons.wikimedia.org/wiki/File:InternetDating.jpg

http://www.surlalunefairytales.com/illustrations/rapunzel/cranera
p3.html

https://commons.wikimedia.org/wiki/File:Palm_fruit_milk_shake.JPG

"CinemaxX Darmstadt 1". Licensed under CC BY-SA 3.0 via Wikimedia Commons - https://commons.wikimedia.org/wiki/File:CinemaxX_Darmstadt_1.JPG#/media/File:CinemaxX_Darmstadt_1.JPG

https://commons.wikimedia.org/wiki/File:Picto_Couple_Dance.png

"おしゃれ帽子 (5507063639)" by bfdingo - Freya & Ellie. Licensed under CC BY-SA 2.0 via Wikimedia Commons - https://commons.wikimedia.org/wiki/File:%E3%81%8A%E3%81%97%E3%82%83%E3%82%8C%E5%B8%BD%E5%AD%90_(5507063639).jpg#/media/File:%E3%81%8A%E3%81%97%E3%82%83%E3%82%8C%E5%B8%BD%E5%AD%90_(5507063639).jpg

"Wikistretnutie 01.07.2005-Thora" by [[:sk:User:{{{1}}}|{{{1}}}]] at the Slovak language Wikipedia. Licensed under CC BY-SA 3.0 via Wikimedia Commons - https://commons.wikimedia.org/wiki/File:Wikistretnutie_01.07.2005-Thora.JPG#/media/File:Wikistretnutie_01.07.2005-Thora.JPG

https://commons.wikimedia.org/wiki/File:Malaysian_playing_golf.jpg

https://commons.wikimedia.org/wiki/File:Ice_skating_rink_in_Bryant_Park.jpg

https://commons.wikimedia.org/wiki/File:Youth_Park_Roller_Skating_Rink.jpg

https://commons.wikimedia.org/wiki/File:SIERRA_CLUB_NATURE_HIKE_-_NARA_-_543233.jpg

https://commons.wikimedia.org/wiki/File:Nilsen-Cultra_vs_China_-_Flickr_-_familymwr.jpg

https://commons.wikimedia.org/wiki/File:Teens_sharing_a_song.jpg

"Victoria, Princess Royal - Romeo meets Juliet" by Victoria, Princess Royal - http://www.royalcollection.org.uk/collection/981276. Licensed under Public Domain via Wikimedia Commons - https://commons.wikimedia.org/wiki/File:Victoria,_Princess_Royal_-_Romeo_meets_Juliet.jpg#/media/File:Victoria,_Princess_Royal_-_Romeo_meets_Juliet.jpg

Chapter Three: Responsibility and Prevention Part I: Avoiding Pitfalls

http://kidshealth.org/teen/

http://psychcentral.com/blog/archives/2013/02/20/signs-of-emotional-abuse/

http://kff.org/womens-health-policy/fact-sheet/sexual-health-of-adolescents-and-young-adults-in-the-united-states/

http://www.hercampus.com/love/relationships/11-worst-gifts-get-your-boyfriend-holidays

http://nypost.com/2013/12/09/the-10-worst-presents-men-get-women-for-the-holidays/

http://www.huffingtonpost.com/2014/11/05/stealing-someones-partner_n_6102094.html

http://www.wikihow.com/Get-Over-Someone-You-Obsess-Over

http://www.evanmarckatz.com/blog/dating-tips-advice/why-don%E2%80%99t-men-hate-being-single-as-much-as-women-do/

http://www.quora.com/Why-are-women-more-keen-on-getting-married-than-men

http://www.ishouldhavesaid.net/2012/01/when-are-you-going-to-find-a-boyfriend-more-answers/

http://www.ishouldhavesaid.net/2012/01/are-you-gay-more-comebacks/

http://www.wikihow.com/Break-Up-with-Someone-You-Love

http://www.usnews.com/news/articles/2012/12/11/scientists-may-have-finally-unlocked-puzzle-of-why-people-are-gay

https://www.washingtonpost.com/news/wonk/wp/2015/03/10/the-u-s-is-still-divided-on-what-causes-homosexuality/

https://en.wikipedia.org/wiki/LGBT_demographics_of_the_United_States

http://www.statista.com/topics/1249/homosexuality/

https://www.washingtonpost.com/news/volokh-conspiracy/wp/2014/07/15/what-percentage-of-the-u-s-population-is-gay-lesbian-or-bisexual/

http://www.kinseyinstitute.org/resources/FAQ.html#Age

http://kidshealth.org/teen/your_mind/relationships/date_rape.html#

http://en.wikipedia.org/wiki/Rape_culture

http://www.teensadvisor.com/teen-dating/being-ready.html

http://thehathorlegacy.com/how-not-to-raise-a-rapist/

http://www.dailymail.co.uk/femail/article-433489/I-seduced-boy-12.html

http://www.babble.com/babble-voices/13-characteristics-of-a-date-rapist-a-list-you-need-to-share/

http://www.chooseresponsibility.org/frequently_asked_questions/

http://www.clarkprosecutor.org/html/domviol/facts.htm

http://pubs.niaaa.nih.gov/publications/AA67/AA67.htm

https://ncadd.org/for-the-media/alcohol-a-drug-information

http://www.drugfreeworld.org/drugfacts.html

http://alcoholrehab.com/drug-addiction/sexual-exploitation-and-substance-abuse/

http://www.thedailybeast.com/articles/2011/02/18/drinking-facts-alcohol-problems-around-the-world.html

http://brown.edu/Student_Services/Health_Services/Health_Education/sexual_health/sexuality/pornography.php

http://en.wikipedia.org/wiki/Pornography_addiction

Illustrations

De Alice's Abenteuer im Wunderland Carroll pic 08" by Lewis Carroll - pdf from gasl.org. Licensed under Public Domain via Wikimedia Commons - http://commons.wikimedia.org/wiki/File:De_Alice%27s_Abenteuer_im_Wunderland_Carroll_pic_08.jpg#/media/File:De_Alice%27s_Abenteuer_im_Wunderland_Carroll_pic_08.jpg https://commons.wikimedia.org/wiki/File:Ducksheep_stuffed_an imal.jpg

https://commons.wikimedia.org/wiki/File:Endust_duster_in_use. jpeg

https://commons.wikimedia.org/wiki/File:Gong-Zappa-Tel-Aviv-2009-10-31-13.jpg

https://commons.wikimedia.org/wiki/File:Napoleon_Hill_holdin g_book_1937.jpg

https://upload.wikimedia.org/wikipedia/commons/d/d0/Leominst er_Museum_-_2014-07-11_-_Andy_Mabbett_-_15.JPG

https://commons.wikimedia.org/wiki/File:Pedometer.jpg

"Boomerang". Licensed under Public Domain via Wikimedia Commons - https: //commons.wikimedia.org/wiki/File:Boomerang.jpg#/media/ File:Boomerang.jpg

https://commons.wikimedia.org/wiki/File:Negligee.jpg

"BCIPodTouch". Licensed under Public Domain via Wikimedia Commons - https://commons.wikimedia.org/wiki/File:BCIPodTouch.JPG #/media/File:BCIPodTouch.JPG

https://commons.wikimedia.org/wiki/File:CAAM30TH.jpg

"Rocky Mountain Views cover" by The Van Noy Inter-State Company - cover of Rocky Mountain Views, published 1917 by The Smith-Brooks Printing Company. Scan by User:Jameslwoodward.. Licensed under Public Domain via Wikimedia Commons - https://commons.wikimedia.org/wiki/File:Rocky_Mountain_ Views_ cover.jpg#/media/File:Rocky_Mountain_Views_cover.jpg

"Martin Van Maele - La Grande Danse macabre des vifs - 34" by Martin van Maële - Illustration de La Grande Danse macabre des vifs. Licensed under Public Domain via Wikimedia Commons - https://commons.wikimedia.org/wiki/File:Martin_Van_Maele_-_La_Grande_Danse_macabre_des_vifs_-_34.jpg#/media/File: Martin_Van_Maele_-_La_Grande_Danse_macabre_des_vifs_-_34.jpg

https://commons.wikimedia.org/wiki/File:Snow-queen.jpg

https://commons.wikimedia.org/wiki/File:The_Marsh_King%27s_Daughter_2_-_Anne_Anderson.jpg

https://commons.wikimedia.org/wiki/File:NOLAMarchItMatters.jpg

https://commons.wikimedia.org/wiki/File:Alcohol_bottles_through_multiprism_filter.jpg

https://commons.wikimedia.org/wiki/File:USMC-100209-M-1998T-001.jpg

https://commons.wikimedia.org/wiki/File:Igle_narkomanov.JPG

https://commons.wikimedia.org/wiki/File:Jen_Su_at_the_Playboy_Magazine_SA_Official_Launch.jpg

https://commons.wikimedia.org/wiki/File:Twilight_stubs.png

https://commons.wikimedia.org/wiki/File:The_real_Alice_in_Wonderland,_Alice_Lindell,_1862.jpg

Chapter Four: Responsibility and Prevention Part II: The Company You Keep – Real and Virtual

http://www.sdcda.org/preventing/protecting-children-online/facts-for-parents.html

http://www.nationalcac.org/prevention/internet-safety-kids.html

http://www.wired.com/2014/08/operation_torpedo/

http://www.makeuseof.com/tag/how-to-remove-false-libelous-information-about-yourself-online/

http://news.yahoo.com/the-11-worst-internet-scams-we-1283163153588278.html

http://www.fraud.org/learn/internet-fraud

https://www.onguardonline.gov/articles/0002-common-online-scams

http://www.nbcnews.com/id/44523031/ns/business-consumer_news/t/how-avoid-nasty-fake-antivirus-scam/#.VrLVOJ16cdU

https://www.scamwatch.gov.au/types-of-scams/unexpected-money/inheritance-scams

https://www.carbuyingtips.com/warranty.htm

http://www.edmunds.com/auto-warranty/third-party-extended-warranty-scams.html

http://www.computerhope.com/issues/ch001045.htm

http://us.norton.com/how-to-be-pirate-free/article

http://www.smartvoter.org/voter/judgecan.html

https://en.wikipedia.org/wiki/Cult

https://en.wikipedia.org/wiki/List_of_religions_and_spiritual_traditions

http://www.apologeticsindex.org/265-who-joins-cults-and-why

Barrett, David V. *The New Believers: Sects, 'Cults' and Alternative Religions*. Cassell. 2003. Print.

Porterfield, Kay Marie. *Straight Talk About Cults*. Cahners Business Information, Inc. 1995. Print.

http://www.christianitytoday.com/iyf/advice/faithqa/what-is-cult.html

http://www.culthelp.info/index.php?option=com_content&task=view&id=15&Itemid=5

http://mediasmarts.ca/online-hate/deconstructing-online-hate

http://www.cultnews.com/2014/10/isis-death-cult-and-internet-brainwashing/

http://cnsnews.com/news/article/patrick-goodenough/al-qaeda-encourages-lone-jihad-attacks-promises-virgins-paradise

http://www.spiritwatch.org/cultmyths.htm

http://articles.sun-sentinel.com/1993-04-20/news/9302070075_1_paul-fatta-cult-member-mass-suicide

http://people.missouristate.edu/michaelcarlie/what_i_learned_about/gangs/getting_out_of_a_gang.htm

https://en.wikiquote.org/wiki/Erhard_Seminars_Training

http://www.watchman.org/index-of-cults-and-religions/

https://en.wikipedia.org/wiki/Landmark_Worldwide

https://en.wikipedia.org/wiki/River_Phoenix

http://jonestown.sdsu.edu/?page_id=35419

http://www.wikihow.com/Leave-a-Cult

http://www.wikihow.com/Avoid-Cults-That-May-Try-to-Convert-You

http://www.linguisticsociety.org/content/how-many-languages-are-there-world

Illustrations

"Computer n screen" by Everaldo Coelho and YellowIcon - All Crystal icons were posted by the author as LGPL on kde-look. Licensed under LGPL via Wikimedia Commons - https://commons.wikimedia.org/wiki/File:Computer_n_screen.svg#/media/File:Computer_n_screen.svg

https://commons.wikimedia.org/wiki/File:Your_Guardian_Angel.jpg

https://commons.wikimedia.org/w/index.php?curid=104136

https://commons.wikimedia.org/wiki/File:Hates_abduction.jpg

By Matthieu Riegler, Wikimedia Commons, CC BY 3.0, https://commons.wikimedia.org/w/index.php?curid=8258135

https://commons.wikimedia.org/wiki/File:Dealing_with_bullies_colored.jpg

By No machine-readable author provided. Skies assumed (based on copyright claims). - No machine-readable source provided. Own work assumed (based on copyright claims)., Public Domain, https://commons.wikimedia.org/w/index.php?curid=2496069

By Photo by one of the Barrow gang - This image is available from the United States Library of Congress's Prints and

Photographs division under the digital ID cph.3c34474.This tag does not indicate the copyright status of the attached work. A normal copyright tag is still required. See Commons:Licensing for more information.العربية | čeština | Deutsch | English | español | فارسی | suomi | français | magyar | italiano | македонски | മലയാളം | Nederlands | polski | português | русский | slovenčina | slovenščina | Türkçe | українська | 中文 | 中文（简体） | 中文（繁體） | +/−, Public Domain, https://commons.wikimedia.org/w/index.php?curid=3109596

By Republican Party (United States) - http://www.gop.com/, Public Domain, https://commons.wikimedia.org/w/index.php?curid=38889019

By David Ball - Original work, CC BY 2.5, https://commons.wikimedia.org/w/index.php?curid=1618965

By Therightclicks - Own work, CC BY-SA 3.0, https://commons.wikimedia.org/w/index.php?curid=9970434

https://commons.wikimedia.org/wiki/File:Libertarian_porcupine_version_2.svg

https://commons.wikimedia.org/wiki/File:Sunflower_(Green_symbol).svg

https://commons.wikimedia.org/wiki/Category:Sow_the_Seeds_of_Victory!#/media/File:Sow_victory_poster_usgovt.gif

https://commons.wikimedia.org/wiki/File:Mevlana_Konya.jpg

"Karnevalswagen Klischee Wirklichkeit 2007" by Jacques Tilly - From the author. Licensed under CC BY 3.0 via Wikimedia Commons - https://commons.wikimedia.org/wiki/File:Karnevalswagen_

Klischee_Wirklichkeit_2007.jpg#/media/File:Karnevalswage n_Klischee_Wirklichkeit_2007.jpg

"Barack Obama and Billy Graham" by The White House from Washington, DC - P042510PS-0042. Licensed under Public Domain via Wikimedia Commons - https://commons.wikimedia.org/wiki/File:Barack_Obama_an d_Billy_Graham.jpg#/media/File:Barack_Obama_and_Billy _Graham.jpg

"Jim Jones, 1977" by Nancy Wong - Own work. Licensed under CC BY-SA 3.0 via Wikimedia Commons - https://commons.wikimedia.org/wiki/File:Jim_Jones,_1977.j pg#/media/File:Jim_Jones,_1977.jpg

"Judgment Bus New Orleans 2011" by Bart Everson - Flickr: Judgment Bus. Licensed under CC BY 2.0 via Wikimedia Commons - https://commons.wikimedia.org/wiki/File:Judgment_Bus_Ne w_Orleans_2011.jpg#/media/File:Judgment_Bus_New_Orle ans_2011.jpg

https://commons.wikimedia.org/wiki/File:The_Manson_Family.j pg

https://commons.wikimedia.org/wiki/File:%D0%A5%D1%80% D0%B0%D0%BC_%D0%92%D1%81%D0%B5%D1%85_ %D0%A0%D0%B5%D0%BB%D0%B8%D0%B3%D0%B8 %D0%B9.JPG

Chapter Five: Responsibility and Prevention Part III: Sexually Transmitted Diseases

http://www.thestdproject.com/std-list/

http://www.cdc.gov/STD/

http://www.nichd.nih.gov/health/topics/stds/conditioninfo/Pages/types.aspx

http://www.ashasexualhealth.org/std-sti/syphilis.html

http://markmanson.net/std-guide

http://www.nlm.nih.gov/medlineplus/medlineplus.html

http://www.webmd.com/hepatitis/

http://en.wikipedia.org/wiki/Hepatitis_B#Prognosis

http://en.wikipedia.org/wiki/Human_papillomavirus

http://www.avert.org/preventing-mother-child-transmission-hiv.htm

http://www.aids.gov/hiv-aids-basics/hiv-aids-101/signs-and-symptoms/

http://www.webmd.com/hepatitis/features/cure

http://www.cdc.gov/parasites/lice/pubic/

http://healthresearchfunding.org/statistics-pubic-lice/

http://www.rightdiagnosis.com/p/pubic_lice/intro.htm

http://www.oliveoilsource.com/article/olive-oil-one-best-ways-combat-head-lice-its-fact

https://www.ndhealth.gov/head-lice/publications/myths_and_facts.pdf

http://www.mayoclinic.org/diseases-conditions/cmv/basics/definition/con-20029514

http://www.medicinenet.com/cytomegalovirus_cmv/article.htm

http://www.cdc.gov/cmv/overview.html

http://www.mayoclinic.org/diseases-conditions/yeast-infection/basics/definition/con-20035129

http://www.healthline.com/health/vaginal-yeast-infection#Causes2

http://www.webmd.com/women/tc/vaginal-yeast-infections-topic-overview

http://www.drugs.com/health-guide/urethritis.html

http://www.drugs.com/health-guide/urethritis.html

http://public.health.oregon.gov/DiseasesConditions/HIVSTDViralHepatitis/SexuallyTransmittedDisease/Pages/fsngu.aspx

http://www.mayoclinic.org/diseases-conditions/urinary-tract-infection/basics/causes/con-20037892

https://en.wikipedia.org/wiki/Lymphogranuloma_venereum

http://www.cdc.gov/std/tg2015/lgv.htm

http://patient.info/doctor/lymphogranuloma-venereum

http://www.ncbi.nlm.nih.gov/pmc/articles/PMC2780057/

http://emedicine.medscape.com/article/176718-treatment

http://www.thestdproject.com/intestinal-parasites-symptoms-signs-and-symptoms-of-stds-and-stis/

http://www.drugs.com/health-guide/giardiasis.html

http://advocatesaz.org/2012/01/03/sti-awareness-intestinal-parasites/#more-2174

https://en.wikipedia.org/wiki/Mycoplasma_genitalium

http://www.ncbi.nlm.nih.gov/pmc/articles/PMC3102684/

http://www.sahealth.sa.gov.au/wps/wcm/connect/public+content/sa+health+internet/health+topics/health+conditions+prevention+and+treatment/infectious+diseases/mycoplasma+genitalium+infection

http://cid.oxfordjournals.org/content/53/suppl_3/S129.full

http://www.drugs.com/health-guide/urethritis.html

http://www.drugs.com/health-guide/urethritis.html

http://public.health.oregon.gov/DiseasesConditions/HIVSTDViralHepatitis/SexuallyTransmittedDisease/Pages/fsngu.aspx

http://www.mayoclinic.org/diseases-conditions/urinary-tract-infection/basics/causes/con-20037892

https://en.wikipedia.org/wiki/Chancroid

http://www.plannedparenthood.org/learn/stds-hiv-safer-sex/chancroid

http://medical-dictionary.thefreedictionary.com/chancroid

http://www.webmd.com/skin-problems-and-treatments/tc/molluscum-contagiosum-topic-overview

http://www.cdc.gov/poxvirus/molluscum-contagiosum/

https://www.gstatic.com/healthricherkp/pdf/molluscum_contagiosum.pdf

https://en.wikipedia.org/wiki/Scabies

http://www.cdc.gov/parasites/scabies/gen_info/faqs.html

http://patient.info/health/scabies-leaflet

http://www.mayoclinic.org/diseases-
    conditions/mononucleosis/basics/definition/con-20021164

https://www.nlm.nih.gov/medlineplus/infectiousmononucleosis.h
    tml

http://www.webmd.com/a-to-z-guides/who-is-affected-by-
    infectious-mononucleosis

http://www.mayoclinic.org/male-yeast-infection/expert-
    answers/faq-20058464

Illustrations

https://commons.wikimedia.org/wiki/File:Human_Immunodefice
    ncy_Virus_-_stylized_rendering.jpg

https://commons.wikimedia.org/wiki/File:Cytomegalovirus_(CM
    V)_Placentitis_(3272294986).jpg

https://commons.wikimedia.org/wiki/File:Herpes_simplex_virus
    _TEM_B82-0474_lores.jpg

https://commons.wikimedia.org/wiki/File:Parasite140131-
    fig1_Capillaria_plectropomi_(Nematoda)_-
    _line_drawings.tif

"Mycoplasma genitalium". Licensed under Public Domain via
    Commons -
    https://commons.wikimedia.org/wiki/File:Mycoplasma_genit
    alium.gif#/media/File:Mycoplasma_genitalium.gif

https://commons.wikimedia.org/wiki/File:Chlamydia_trachomati
    s_Bacteria_and_the_PmpD_Protein_(6829956633).jpg

"EM of pap virus, 2C basal tissue grafted to mouse" by PhD Dre
- http://en.wikipedia.org/wiki/Image:EM_of_pap_virus%2C_b asal_tissue_grafted_to_mouse.jpg. Licensed under CC BY-SA 3.0 via Wikimedia Commons - https://commons.wikimedia.org/wiki/File:EM_of_pap_virus,_2C_basal_tissue_grafted_to_mouse.jpg#/media/File:EM_of_pap_virus,_2C_basal_tissue_grafted_to_mouse.jpg

"Body lice" by Janice Harney Carr, Center for Disease Control - This media comes from the Centers for Disease Control and Prevention's Public Health Image Library (PHIL), with identification number #9217.Note: Not all PHIL images are public domain; be sure to check copyright status and credit authors and content providers.English | Slovenščina | +/−. Licensed under Public Domain via Wikimedia Commons - https://commons.wikimedia.org/wiki/File:Body_lice.jpg#/media/File:Body_lice.jpg

"Pediculus humanus development numberedblackwhite" by Pediculus_humanus_development_numbered.png: *Pediculus_humanus_development.jpg: CDCderivative work: B kimmel (talk)derivative work: B kimmel (talk) - Pediculus_humanus_development_numbered.png. Licensed under Public Domain via Wikimedia Commons - https://commons.wikimedia.org/wiki/File:Pediculus_humanus_development_numberedblackwhite.png#/media/File:Pediculus_humanus_development_numberedblackwhite.png

"Hepatitis B virus 01" by This media comes from the Centers for Disease Control and Prevention's Public Health Image Library (PHIL), with identification number #270.Note: Not all PHIL images are public domain; be sure to check copyright status and credit authors and content providers.English | Slovenščina | +/−O*btained from the CDC Public Health Image Library.Image credit: CDC/Dr. Erskine Palmer (PHIL #270), 1981.http://images.encarta.msn.com/xrefmedia/sharemed/targets/images/

"Sarcoptes scabei 2" by Kalumet - de.wikipedia. Licensed under CC BY-SA 3.0 via Wikimedia Commons - https://commons.wikimedia.org/wiki/File:Sarcoptes_scabei_2.jpg#/media/File:Sarcoptes_scabei_2.jpg

https://commons.wikimedia.org/wiki/File:Infectious_Mononucleosis_3.jpg

https://commons.wikimedia.org/wiki/File:Syphilis_Bacteria_(16842837731).jpg
"Haemophilus ducreyi 01". Licensed under Public Domain via Wikimedia Commons - https://commons.wikimedia.org/wiki/File:Haemophilus_ducreyi_01.jpg#/media/File:Haemophilus_ducreyi_01.jpg

https://commons.wikimedia.org/wiki/File:Vaginose-G15.jpg

"Candidiasis (5494228352)" by Yale Rosen from USA - CandidiasisUploaded by CFCF. Licensed under CC BY-SA 2.0 via Wikimedia Commons - https://commons.wikimedia.org/wiki/File:Candidiasis_(5494228352).jpg#/media/File:Candidiasis_(5494228352).jpg

https://commons.wikimedia.org/wiki/File:Neutrophils_phagocytizing_bacteria.jpg

https://commons.wikimedia.org/wiki/File:Blausen_0732_PID-Sites.png

https://commons.wikimedia.org/wiki/File:Theodor_Kittelsen_-_Skovtrold_(1899).jpg

Chapter Six: Responsibility and Prevention Part IV: Birth Control

http://womensissues.about.com/od/datingandsex/a/10-Arguments-For-Abstinence-Pros-And-Cons-Of-The-Abstinence-Debate-Part-I.htm

http://www.plannedparenthood.org/health-topics/birth-control/withdrawal-pull-out-method-4218.htm

http://www.contracept.org/none.php

http://www.historiann.com/2012/03/13/lysol-americas-most-destructive-and-least-effective-form-of-contraception/

http://www.plannedparenthood.org/health-topics/birth-control-4211.htm

http://www.plannedparenthood.org/files/PPFA/history_bc_methods.pdf

http://www.sciencedaily.com/releases/2007/02/070221065200.htm

http://www.ask.com/question/advantages-and-disadvantages-of-male-sterilization

http://www.ask.com/question/advantages-and-disadvantages-of-male-sterilization

http://americanpregnancy.org/preventingpregnancy/male-condom/

http://americanpregnancy.org/preventingpregnancy/female-condom/

http://en.wikipedia.org/wiki/Spermicide

http://www.science20.com/news_articles/multiple_abortions_increase_risks_subsequent_delivered_babies-93475

http://money.cnn.com/2014/08/18/pf/child-cost/

http://www.babymed.com/getting-pregnant/what-are-the-odds-conceiving-conception

https://en.wikipedia.org/wiki/Criminal_transmission_of_HIV

http://projects.propublica.org/tables/penalties

http://www.shouselaw.com/nevada/intentional-hiv-transmission.html

Illustrations

https://commons.wikimedia.org/wiki/File:OldWomanWho-Open.JPG

https://commons.wikimedia.org/wiki/File:MGD88FrogNunPriest.jpg

"Female anatomy frontal". Licensed under Public Domain via Wikimedia Commons -
"Vasectomy" by Rhcastilhos -
http://commons.wikimedia.org/wiki/File:Vasectomia.jpg.
Licensed under CC0 via Wikimedia Commons -
https://commons.wikimedia.org/wiki/File:Female_anatomy_frontal.png#/media/File:Female_anatomy_frontal.png

https://commons.wikimedia.org/wiki/File:Vasectomy.jpg#/media/File:Vasectomy.jpg

https://commons.wikimedia.org/wiki/File:Implanon_03.jpg

https://commons.wikimedia.org/wiki/File:Koperspiraal.jpg

https://commons.wikimedia.org/wiki/File:Mother_breast_feeding _baby.jpg

https://commons.wikimedia.org/wiki/File:Prikpil.JPG

https://commons.wikimedia.org/wiki/Vaginal_ring#/media/File: NuvaRing_in_hand.jpg

https://commons.wikimedia.org/wiki/Category:Birth_control#/m edia/File:Lutera_(Birth_Control_Pills).jpg

https://commons.wikimedia.org/wiki/File:BirthControlPatch.JPG

https://commons.wikimedia.org/wiki/File:Contraceptive_diaphra gm.jpg

https://commons.wikimedia.org/wiki/File:Contraceptive_sponge, _United_Kingdom,_1901-1930_Wellcome_L0065290.jpg

https://commons.wikimedia.org/wiki/File:Pdgd.jpg

https://commons.wikimedia.org/wiki/Category:Female_condoms

https://commons.wikimedia.org/wiki/Category:Male_condoms#/ media/File:Condom_rolled.jpg

https://commons.wikimedia.org/wiki/File:Condom,_glow_in_the _dark.jpg

https://commons.wikimedia.org/wiki/Category:Birth_control#/m edia/File:Abstinence_during_fertile_period.png

April, With Intriguing Books and Suffering Withdrawal" by Name invalid - Own work. Licensed under Public Domain via Wikimedia Commons - http://commons.wikimedia.org/wiki/File:April,_With_Intrigu ing_Books_and_Suffering_Withdrawal.jpg#/media/File:Apri l,_With_Intriguing_Books_and_Suffering_Withdrawal.jpg

https://commons.wikimedia.org/wiki/File:Globulka.jpg

https://commons.wikimedia.org/wiki/File:Cape_cervicale.jpg

Chapter Seven: Make Romance + Finance = Transcen-Dance

http://en.wikipedia.org/wiki/Money

http://www.investopedia.com/university/beginner/beginner2.asp#axzz1yNC6V2sB

http://en.wikipedia.org/wiki/Personal_budget

https://www.nerdwallet.com/blog/credit-cards/credit-card-basics-high-school-students/

http://moneytalks4teens.ucanr.edu/faq.cfm?faq=176

https://smartasset.com/credit-cards/what-is-a-good-debt-to-income-ratio

http://www.clearpoint.org/blog/what-is-a-good-debt-to-income-ratio-anyway/

http://www.ckfraud.org/penalties.html

http://parade.condenast.com/292912/viannguyen/the-average-cost-of-a-wedding-in-each-region-of-the-u-s/

https://www.healthcare.gov/medicaid-chip/getting-medicaid-chip/

http://en.wikipedia.org/wiki/Life_insurance

https://www.trustedchoice.com/renters-insurance/coverage-rate-cost/

http://www.learnvest.com/knowledge-center/how-much-do-funerals-cost/

http://www.wikihow.com/Write-a-Living-Will

Illustrations

"000dd556 medium" by Dik Browne - Gilberton. Licensed under Public Domain via Wikimedia Commons - http://commons.wikimedia.org/wiki/File:000dd556_medium.jpeg#/media/File:000dd556_medium.jpeg

https://commons.wikimedia.org/wiki/File:Arbetsmiljo_(6).jpg

https://upload.wikimedia.org/wikipedia/commons/6/68/Auto_Mechanic.jpg

"VentureTimeline". Licensed under CC BY-SA 3.0 via Wikimedia Commons - https://commons.wikimedia.org/wiki/File:VentureTimeline.png#/media/File:VentureTimeline.png

https://commons.wikimedia.org/wiki/File:Commonwealth_Bank_of_Australia_-_old_savings_passbook.jpg

https://commons.wikimedia.org/wiki/File:US-$10000-Certificate_of_Deposit-1875_(Proof).jpg

https://commons.wikimedia.org/wiki/File:Money_market_fund.png

"US-Funded Loan of 1891-$20,000 (face only)" by National Museum of American History - Image by Godot13. Licensed under Public Domain via Wikimedia Commons - https://commons.wikimedia.org/wiki/File:US-Funded_Loan_of_1891-$20,000_(face_only).jpg#/media/File:US-Funded_Loan_of_1891-$20,000_(face_only).jpg

"DJIA 2000s graph (log)" by
DJIA_historical_graph_to_jan09_(log).svg:
*DJIA_historical_graph_(log).svg: The original uploader
was Lalala666 at English Wikipediaderivative work:
DavidRF (talk)derivative work: DavidRF (talk) - DJIA
historical graph (log).svg. Licensed under Public Domain via
Wikimedia Commons -
https://commons.wikimedia.org/wiki/File:DJIA_2000s_graph
_(log).svg#/media/File:DJIA_2000s_graph_(log).svg

https://commons.wikimedia.org/wiki/File:Asset_class_wise_hold
ings_in_mutual_fund_industry.png

https://commons.wikimedia.org/wiki/File:United_States_Depart
ment_of_Labor_-_Strategic_Plan_Fiscal_Years_2011-
2016.pdf

https://commons.wikimedia.org/wiki/File:Pigeon_Nest_Egg.jpg

https://commons.wikimedia.org/wiki/File:Annuity_0004.pdf

"Seattle uitgaven 2014" by Supercarwaar - Own work; data
evidently from Mayor McGinn's 2014 Proposed Budget,
page 6, presented on September 23, 2013. (The numbers
match those given at [1].). Licensed under CC BY-SA 3.0 via
Wikimedia Commons -
https://commons.wikimedia.org/wiki/File:Seattle_uitgaven_2
014.png#/media/File:Seattle_uitgaven_2014.png

https://commons.wikimedia.org/wiki/File:Check_Book.jpg

By Lotus Head from Johannesburg, Gauteng, South Africa -
sxc.hu, CC BY-SA 3.0,
https://commons.wikimedia.org/w/index.php?curid=99950

"Payday loan shop window" by Gregory F. Maxwell
<gmaxwell@gmail.com> PGP:0xB0413BFA - Own work
(Original caption: "By Uploader"). Licensed under GFDL
1.2 via Wikimedia Commons -

https://commons.wikimedia.org/wiki/File:Payday_loan_shop_window.jpg#/media/File:Payday_loan_shop_window.jpg

"Санкт-Петербург 2010 (0040)" by S URALA - Own work. Licensed under CC BY-SA 3.0 via Wikimedia Commons - https://commons.wikimedia.org/wiki/File:%D0%A1%D0%B0%D0%BD%D0%BA%D1%82-%D0%9F%D0%B5%D1%82%D0%B5%D1%80%D0%B1%D1%83%D1%80%D0%B3_2010_(0040).jpg#/media/File:%D0%A1%D0%B0%D0%BD%D0%BA%D1%82-%D0%9F%D0%B5%D1%82%D0%B5%D1%80%D0%B1%D1%83%D1%80%D0%B3_2010_(0040).jpg

https://commons.wikimedia.org/wiki/File:Yellow_Mustang_Car.JPG

"Damon Sacks" by Damonsacks - Own work. Licensed under CC BY-SA 3.0 via Wikimedia Commons - https://commons.wikimedia.org/wiki/File:Damon_Sacks.JPG#/media/File:Damon_Sacks.JPG

https://upload.wikimedia.org/wikipedia/commons/5/52/Apartment_hotel_in_Kilpisj%C3%A4rvi.jpg

"Chart of a life insurance" by Justin Arndt - https://sites.google.com/site/moblopedia/life-insurance/Chart_of_a_life_insurance.jpg. Licensed under CC BY-SA 3.0 via Wikimedia Commons - https://commons.wikimedia.org/wiki/File:Chart_of_a_life_insurance.jpg#/media/File:Chart_of_a_life_insurance.jpg

"Western Necropolis - geograph.org.uk - 57975" by Chris Upson. Licensed under CC BY-SA 2.0 via Wikimedia Commons - https://commons.wikimedia.org/wiki/File:Western_Necropolis_-_geograph.org.uk_-_57975.jpg#/media/File:Western_Necropolis_-_geograph.org.uk_-_57975.jpg

https://commons.wikimedia.org/wiki/File:Health_reform_rally_-_Seattle_-_2009-09-03_-_counterdemonstrators_02.jpg

https://commons.wikimedia.org/wiki/File:The_prodigals_nurse,_or_modern_heir_LCCN2002719531.jpg

"Gold-D" by The original uploader was Lvtalon at English WikipediaLater versions were uploaded by Chisholm4 at en.wikipedia. - Transferred from en.wikipedia to Commons.. Licensed under CC BY-SA 3.0 via Wikimedia Commons - https://commons.wikimedia.org/wiki/File:Gold-D.jpg#/media/File:Gold-D.jpg

Chapter Eight: Tomorrow is not Promised You, But...

http://www.religioustolerance.org/chr_dira.htm

http://divorcescience.org/2012/06/29/351/

http://usatoday30.usatoday.com/news/health/wellness/marriage/story/2011-08-25/Marriage-divorce-rates-higher-in-the-South-lower-in-Northeast/50126268/1

http://patch.com/georgia/marietta/the-top-10-reasons-marriages-end-in-divorce_14370092

http://www.yourtango.com/experts/yourtango-experts/top-causes-divorce-expert

http://divorcesupport.about.com/od/isdivorcethesolution/a/Three-Major-Causes-Of-Divorce.htm

http://www.divorce.usu.edu/files/uploads/lesson3.pdf

http://www.scienceofrelationships.com/home/2012/4/19/the-top-20-most-desired-personality-traits-in-a-future-spous.html

http://www.truthaboutdeception.com/lying-and-deception/what-lovers-lie-about.html

http://madamenoire.com/192697/are-you-marriage-material-7-signs-you-may-not-make-a-good-wife/2/

http://thoughtcatalog.com/derek-marshall/2013/11/40-people-on-the-worst-trait-a-significant-other-can-have/

http://love.allwomenstalk.com/things-to-discuss-with-him-before-marriage

http://www.huffingtonpost.com/2013/05/26/sex-before-marriage_n_3333073.html

http://www.debate.org/opinions/is-sex-before-marriage-okay

http://www.webmd.com/sex-relationships/news/20101227/theres-benefits-in-delaying-sex-until-marriage

http://discoveringtherealme.wikispaces.com/11+-+Should+You+Have+Sex+Before+Marriage%3F

http://marriage.about.com/od/cohabitation/qt/cohabfacts.htm

http://www.sdflaw.com/news-media/shifting-gender-roles-and-it-s-impact-on-divorce/

http://iussp.org/sites/default/files/event_call_for_papers/IUSSP%20Extended%20abstract%20divorce.pdf

http://www.eharmony.com/blog/2011/10/05/when-dating-how-long-do-you-wait-for-the-ring/#.U5iDH8JOVjo

http://en.wikipedia.org/wiki/Change_in_personality_over_a_lifetime

http://webcenters.netscape.compuserve.com/love/package.jsp?name=fte/idealagetomarry/idealagetomarry

http://www.gallup.com/poll/23404/ideal-age-marriage-women-men.aspx

http://www.friendsandfamilyforum.com/showthread.php?t=5398

Illustrations

http://savannahnow.com/bluffton-news/2012-07-04/brothers-grimm-fairy-tale-trivia

https://commons.wikimedia.org/wiki/File:Hourglass_drawing.svg

"Communication shannon-weaver2" by Einar Faanes - Own work. Licensed under CC BY-SA 3.0 via Wikimedia Commons - https://commons.wikimedia.org/wiki/File:Communication_shannon-weaver2.svg#/media/File:Communication_shannon-weaver2.svg

"Axolotlpainting" by Orizatriz - Own work. Licensed under CC BY-SA 3.0 via Wikimedia Commons - https://commons.wikimedia.org/wiki/File:Axolotlpainting.jpg#/media/File:Axolotlpainting.jpg

https://commons.wikimedia.org/wiki/File:Compassion-Logo.png

"Raja Ravi Varma, At the Bath" by Raja Ravi Varma - http://www.museumsyndicate.com/item.php?item=25455. Licensed under Public Domain via Wikimedia Commons - https://commons.wikimedia.org/wiki/File:Raja_Ravi_Varma,_At_the_Bath.jpg#/media/File:Raja_Ravi_Varma,_At_the_Bath.jpg

"Alfred E. Neumann" by unknown (not relevant to copyright status) - Image from

http://community.webshots.com/photo/304039856/30404176
8aZxySa#. Licensed under Public Domain via Wikimedia
Commons -
https://commons.wikimedia.org/wiki/File:Alfred_E._Neuma
nn.jpg#/media/File:Alfred_E._Neumann.jpg

https://commons.wikimedia.org/wiki/File:Handshake_icon_GRE
EN-BLUE.svg

"Heckel Hindu Kush 3" by Vilém Heckel -
http://www.vilemheckel.cz/. Licensed under CC BY-SA 3.0
via Wikimedia Commons -
https://commons.wikimedia.org/wiki/File:Heckel_Hindu_Ku
sh_3.jpg#/media/File:Heckel_Hindu_Kush_3.jpg

https://commons.wikimedia.org/wiki/File:Thank_You!.jpg

https://commons.wikimedia.org/wiki/File:Greed_1924_poster.jp
g

"A secret moment" by Unknown - Bukowskis. Licensed under
Public Domain via Wikimedia Commons -
https://commons.wikimedia.org/wiki/File:A_secret_moment.
jpg#/media/File:A_secret_moment.jpg

"Rage face" by Smurfy - Own work. Licensed under Public
Domain via Wikimedia Commons -
https://commons.wikimedia.org/wiki/File:Rage_face.png#/m
edia/File:Rage_face.png

https://commons.wikimedia.org/wiki/File:The_English_Councill
ors.JPG

https://commons.wikimedia.org/wiki/File:Street_Art_-
_Green_Monster.jpg

"1916MomusPinocchio" by Not credited - 1916 printing via [1].
Licensed under Public Domain via Wikimedia Commons -

https://commons.wikimedia.org/wiki/File:1916MomusPinocchio.jpg#/media/File:1916MomusPinocchio.jpg

https://commons.wikimedia.org/wiki/File:Alcohol_bottles_through_multiprism_filter.jpg

https://commons.wikimedia.org/wiki/File:USMC-100209-M-1998T-001.jpg

https://commons.wikimedia.org/wiki/File:Igle_narkomanov.JPG

https://commons.wikimedia.org/wiki/File:The_Spoiled_Child_by_Meadows.png

"Desidia - The Seven Deadly Sins - Pieter Brueghel" by Pieter Brueghel - http://gnozis.info/?q=node/2792. Licensed under Public Domain via Wikimedia Commons - https://commons.wikimedia.org/wiki/File:Desidia_-_The_Seven_Deadly_Sins_-_Pieter_Brueghel.png#/media/File:Desidia_-_The_Seven_Deadly_Sins_-_Pieter_Brueghel.png

"The Eyes of the Antisocials" by Bill Mehalus - Own work. Licensed under CC BY-SA 3.0 via Wikimedia Commons - https://commons.wikimedia.org/wiki/File:The_Eyes_of_the_Antisocials.jpg#/media/File:The_Eyes_of_the_Antisocials.jpg

https://commons.wikimedia.org/wiki/File:Lucille_Ball_and_Desi_Arnaz_at_home_1947.jpg

"Hugo Kauffmann Kinder mit Wagen 1906" by Hugo Kauffmann - Dorotheum. Licensed under Public Domain via Wikimedia Commons - https://commons.wikimedia.org/wiki/File:Hugo_Kauffmann_Kinder_mit_Wagen_1906.jpg#/media/File:Hugo_Kauffmann_Kinder_mit_Wagen_1906.jpg

227

"Francesco Hayez 008" by Francesco Hayez - The Yorck
    Project: 10.000 Meisterwerke der Malerei. DVD-ROM,
    2002. ISBN 3936122202. Distributed by DIRECTMEDIA
    Publishing GmbH. Official, high definition zoomable
    version.. Licensed under Public Domain via Wikimedia
    Commons -
    https://commons.wikimedia.org/wiki/File:Francesco_Hayez_
    008.jpg#/media/File:Francesco_Hayez_008.jpg

https://commons.wikimedia.org/wiki/File:Work_and_leisure.jpg

"Dunce (7885704332)" by Wayne Wilkinson - DunceUploaded
    by AlbertHerring. Licensed under CC BY 2.0 via Wikimedia
    Commons -
    https://commons.wikimedia.org/wiki/File:Dunce_(78857043
    32).jpg#/media/File:Dunce_(7885704332).jpg

"Mutual Life levensverz.-lijfrente" by Unknown -
    www.geheugenvannederland.nl. Licensed under Public
    Domain via Wikimedia Commons -
    https://commons.wikimedia.org/wiki/File:Mutual_Life_leven
    sverz.-lijfrente.jpg#/media/File:Mutual_Life_levensverz.-
    lijfrente.jpg

"The Munsters 1964" by CBS Television - eBay itemphoto
    frontphoto back. Licensed under Public Domain via
    Wikimedia Commons -
    https://commons.wikimedia.org/wiki/File:The_Munsters_196
    4.JPG#/media/File:The_Munsters_1964.JPG

"Bierstadt Albert The Golden Gate" by Albert Bierstadt -
    forum.netfotograf.com. Licensed under Public Domain via
    Wikimedia Commons -
    https://commons.wikimedia.org/wiki/File:Bierstadt_Albert_T
    he_Golden_Gate.jpg#/media/File:Bierstadt_Albert_The_Gol
    den_Gate.jpg

References Illustration

https://commons.wikimedia.org/wiki/File:A_man_in_a_heavy_cl oak_and_hat_is_reading_a_large_book_which_Wellcome_V 0040724.jpg

www.ingramcontent.com/pod-product-compliance
Lightning Source LLC
Chambersburg PA
CBHW071340280526
45787CB00001B/155